THE dairy-free & gluten-free KITCHEN

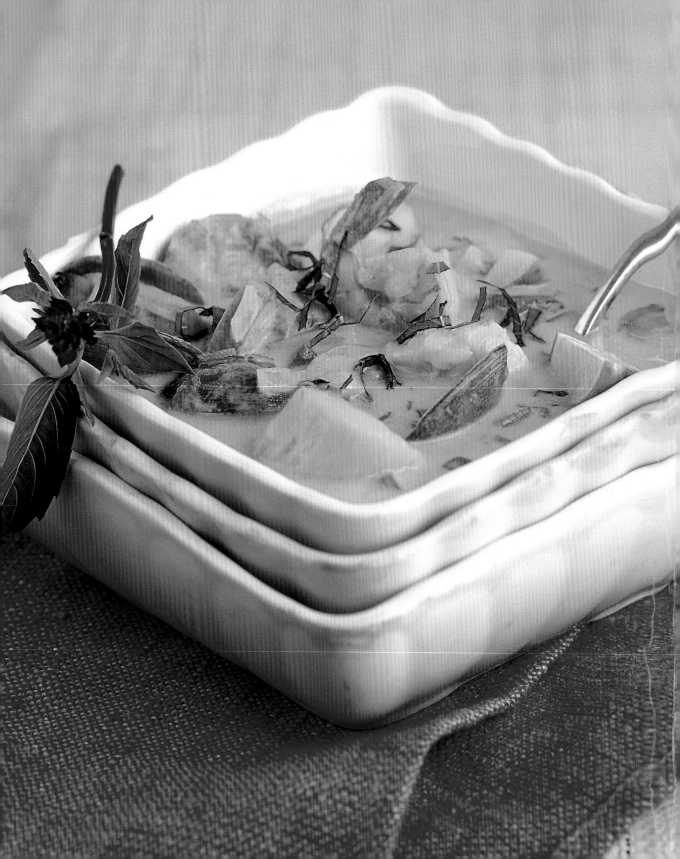

the dairy-free & gluten-free kitchen

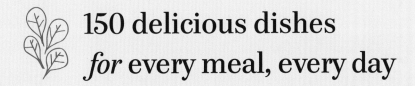 150 delicious dishes
for every meal, every day

Denise Jardine

Photography by Caroline Kopp *and* Erin Kunkel

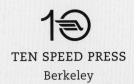

TEN SPEED PRESS

Berkeley

This book is dedicated in loving memory of

my father, Sava Dragisich, whose love transcends time.

It is also dedicated to my mother, Mary,

for nourishing my dreams.

contents

acknowledgments

I could not have written this book without the contributions and support of many talented individuals. My heartfelt thanks to four amazing chefs—Marc Rubenstein, Gerard Rodriguez, Marc, and Maureen Kellond—for their recipe contributions, enthusiasm, and culinary excellence. My sincere appreciation to Chad Lott—a talented writer in his own right—for his manuscript contributions. Thanks to Jennifer Lo for working her magic and creating my website. Thanks also to Amy Vig, Pam Savin, Leanne Valenti, and Linda Frandsen for recipe testing and evaluation. Additional thanks to Norma Quon, Matthew Lederman, MD, Alona Pulde, MD, and Jeff Novick, MS, RD, for their expertise. Also many thanks to the Sarno brothers, Chad and Derek—two inspiring chefs. Working with each of you is an honor and pleasure.

I am immensely grateful to my editor Veronica Randall, art director Toni Tajima, copyeditor Molly Jackel, and production manager Serena Sigona for their expertise and hard work. Thank you also to photographer Erin Kunkel and stylist Erin Quon for the new photography in the second edition.

I must also acknowledge the special people in my life who gave me emotional support and contributed directly and indirectly throughout the development of the recipes and accompanying text. My chief taster and most constructive critic also happens to be my husband Robert. His unwavering encouragement and objective feedback were invaluable to me. He is my life's love and champion.

More personal thanks to Drs. Robert and Nick Stojanovich for hours of insightful conversations. My loving thanks to Linda Cloonan, Annamaria Delgado, Suzanne Allen, and Barbara Ryan for sharing in my journey and cheering me on, no matter what. Also, my deepest thanks to my family past for teaching me how to grow and prepare food with old world sensibilities. And thanks to my family present Nick and Dorothy Dragisich, sissy Marsha van Dongeren, Barry and Bruce Savin, Mark and Teresa Reculin, Andrea Arbore, Bill, Richard, and Susan Jardine, and our dear friends Paul and Lesa Martin, Matt and Jody Friedman, Jim and Mary Fritz, and Steve and Pat Wuthrich for their encouragement, laughter, and sharing in many a marvelous meal.

And last but not least to each of you seeking wellness through my classes, lectures, or this cookbook. You have inspired me to continue doing what I love—thank you.

preface

If you subscribe to the philosophy that life is a marathon and not a sprint, then you will understand why this book came to be.

When I wrote *Recipes for Dairy-Free Living* in 2001, it was almost like a sprint to the finish line of a race to help myself and others deal with a long list of health issues related to dairy food intolerance and allergies. Judging from its popularity over the past ten years, *Recipes for Dairy-Free Living* has resonated with thousands of readers around the world who suffer from health problems related to dairy foods in their diets.

However, a marathoner doesn't stop when the first milestone of the race has been achieved. Instead, a second wind drives the runner onward. My second wind came in the form of continued self-discovery and expanded knowledge about the food-health connection. The next part of my food-health marathon was to pursue a formal education in nutrition, including culinary training on ingredients and techniques to maximize the nutritional value of the food we eat. I was so enthusiastic about the health benefits of a natural, whole-food diet that I became a teacher to students pursuing a nutritional-based culinary career.

Through the course of my training and teaching, I came to realize that many people's dietary health problems (including my own) were not solely the result of dairy foods. In fact, the statistics support the fact that many people who have problems with dairy also suffer from health issues related to gluten products. As awareness of the gluten-health connection has increased in recent years, the number of people formally diagnosed with health problems caused by gluten in their diets has also increased dramatically.

To further my passion for helping others overcome their diet-related health issues, I joined Whole Foods Market® as the Community Healthy Eating Specialist at my hometown store. As a lecturer and in-store culinary guide, I gained first-hand experience helping others cope with the difficulty of implementing dietary changes for themselves, or a family member, after being diagnosed with a disease or condition for which diet was a contributing factor. The relief that customers always displayed upon realizing that healthy and delicious dairy-free and gluten-free food alternatives were readily available was heart warming and gratifying. I received tremendous feedback about the health improvements that dietary modifications were having on people's lives.

Along with the practical feedback on the positive health impacts of dietary changes, I was also receiving on-the-job training about the health benefits of a whole-food, plant-based, healthy fat and nutrient rich diet. There is overwhelming evidence that these dietary improvements directly contribute to health benefits, such as lowering the risk of cardio-vascular disease, diabetes, and obesity.

Based on these experiences, this follow-up book to *Recipes for Dairy-Free Living* began to take shape in my mind. I could see the growing need for a book that focuses not only on eliminating dairy foods but gluten as well, including identifying other food allergens. And I came to learn that these dietary changes should not be the cause of angst and despair. Today, the list of dairy and gluten substitute products is vast and growing every day. So this book is based on the rallying cry I always use with my readers and clients facing the challenge of dietary changes—"It's not about the foods you *can't* have, it's about the wonderful foods you *can* have!" And, as a second but extremely important feature, the recipes in this book have been created with the objective of minimizing unnecessary refined oils, refined sweeteners, and sodium without sacrificing flavor or the satisfaction of the dishes presented.

Just as cheering supporters bolster the marathoner, this book was written because of the many wonderful people who were an inspiration to me. I would like to thank all of the readers of *Recipes for Dairy-Free Living* for their thoughtful feedback and suggestions for recipes, and Bauman College for providing me with a comprehensive educational foundation in whole-food nutrition. I also thank Whole Foods Market® for the opportunity to connect with customers, members of the medical profession, and the community at large. This interaction over the past decade has provided valuable knowledge and input that is a cornerstone of this book.

introduction

Since the first edition of Recipes for Dairy-Free Living *there has been a growing awareness and diagnosis of food intolerances, sensitivities, and allergies.*

Increasingly, people have been looking for alternative ways to eat the foods they love without experiencing the ill side effects. Many individuals who experience health issues related to dairy food consumption have found that wheat and gluten are also contributing factors, myself not withstanding. Although I had discovered my dairy allergy, it wasn't until several years later that I learned I was also intolerant to wheat and gluten. To better understand what it means to be gluten intolerant and eliminate it from your diet, I've added a section on gluten to the introduction that addresses this growing concern and its impact on diet-related health issues.

In this edition, each recipe is not only dairy-free but also 100 percent wheat- and gluten-free! But I didn't stop there. Recognizing that many people who experience food intolerances may also face multiple food allergies, I've included at the top of each recipe, a coding system that indicates other common allergens the recipe is free of. **If you see an asterisk next to an ingredient, it's simply alerting you that the ingredient may be replaced with other options. For example, if you see an asterisk next to soy yogurt* in an ingredients list, and you have a sensitivity to soy products, this indicates that soy yogurt can be replaced with rice or almond yogurt to make the recipe soy-free.**

Furthermore, each recipe has been reformulated to reduce unnecessary oils and refined sweeteners without compromising flavor. The expanded Basics section is the backbone for many of the recipes in this book and is where you will find the master gluten-free flour mix (page 172), instructions for making your own nondairy nut milk (page 173), and nut cheese (page 175). You will also find new recipes in every chapter, photos for inspiration, and an updated listing of manufacturers, distributors, and other resources.

The Dairy-Free & Gluten-Free Kitchen provides the basic information you need to manage your dairy- and gluten-free decisions and offers a collection of delicious recipes—prepared with accessible ingredients—that will make implementing a dairy- and gluten-free diet effortless.

I'd like to extend my sincere appreciation to all of my readers and clients for sharing your food intolerance discoveries over the years—each of you has given me the inspiration for updating and revising *Recipes for Dairy-Free Living* and bringing you this second edition. Thank you and enjoy!

Understanding Dairy Issues

Dairy products and their isolated constituents come in many forms and are in more foods than you might realize. The extracted protein, fat, and sugar from dairy have many different uses in food manufacturing and are used to lend texture, structure, and flavor to so many everyday foods. Beyond the obvious items in the dairy case, many other products contain dairy in the form of lactose or milk proteins. One example is a dairy protein called casein that is often added to milk-alternative cheeses to enable the cheese to melt. In addition to various processed food items, dairy components are also used in pharmaceutical drugs sold both over the counter and by prescription. So the first step in implementing a dairy-free lifestyle is to have a basic understanding of what dairy is and how it can affect us.

Lactose Intolerance

Although the terms *lactose intolerance* and *dairy allergy* are often used interchangeably, they engage very different body processes. Lactose is milk sugar, a carbohydrate, which occurs naturally in the milk of animals. Many people are intolerant to milk products because they lack the enzyme called lactase. This enzyme, found in the gastrointestinal tract, is critical in the digestion of lactose. If the lactase enzyme is missing or depleted, the gastrointestinal tract cannot adequately break down the milk sugar, leading to a wide variety of symptoms. Individuals experiencing this are described as being *lactose intolerant*.

The symptoms of lactose intolerance can vary greatly from one individual to the next as well as varying within the individual. They include, but are not limited to, stomach cramps, bloating, flatulence, and diarrhea. It's difficult to estimate how many people are lactose intolerant. However, it is estimated that up to fifty million Americans suffer from some form of dairy intolerance. The condition encompasses many ethnic groups; age also plays a major role in the ability to tolerate dairy products. As we mature, our body's ability to produce the lactase enzyme in our gastrointestinal tract begins to diminish. That is why lactose intolerance can intensify with age. Tolerance is dependent upon the amount of lactase in each individual's system and the amount of dairy products ingested at any given time. Think of it this way: If you have a limited amount of lactase enzyme in your gastrointestinal tract and you ingest limited amounts of dairy, your body may be able to break the lactose down on its own. However, if you have a limited amount of lactase enzyme available and you ingest moderate to high amounts of dairy, you will have exceeded your body's capacity to digest the lactose and thus will experience symptoms.

Unfortunately, there is no way to establish what constitutes limited, moderate, and high dairy intake, because it is completely individualized. To some people, limited amounts of dairy can translate to milk on their cereal in the morning, yogurt in the afternoon, and pasta with Parmesan cheese for dinner. For others this amount of dairy would be considered high or excessive. And some people could tolerate this amount of dairy only if they avoided dairy products entirely for the next several days.

Many people who are strictly lactose intolerant can avoid problems simply by taking a dairy digestive aid. These digestive aids are widely available and can be purchased over the counter at supermarkets, drugstores, and specialty stores. The amount of lactase enzyme you will require will depend on how much dairy you ingest and how much lactase is already present in your gastrointestinal tract. Select a product that has the right amount of FCC lactase units to complement your digestive tract. For example, when comparing various products I found that the suggested dosage could vary drastically from one product to the next, with one brand containing 9,000 FCC lactase units per caplet and another containing only 1,000.

Milk Proteins and Allergy

Milk proteins come in many different forms, several with names that are difficult to pronounce. The important thing is to be able to recognize them when they appear on a label. The main ones to look for are casein and whey, but proteins can also be identified as hydrolysates, caseinates, lactalbumin, and lactoglobulin. All of these are milk proteins.

As with the symptoms of lactose intolerance, reactions to milk proteins can vary greatly from one individual to the next. Reaction to milk proteins is regarded as a food or dairy allergy. It is important to understand that a food allergy triggers an immune system response to compounds, in this case proteins, in an offending food. It is caused by an allergic antibody called IgE (Immunoglobulin E). However, it is significant to note that it is possible to be both lactose intolerant and develop a food allergy to dairy proteins.

Symptoms of dairy allergy tend to range in severity from digestive issues including: stomach cramps, bloating, flatulence, diarrhea, constipation, bleeding from the bowel, rectal fissures, and itching, to respiratory problems, such as asthma, sinus and lung congestion, ear aches, itchy and watery eyes, skin rash, hives, and eczema. And possible behavioral problems, including migraine headaches, fatigue, brain fog, irritability, and anxiety. If you suspect that you may have a dairy allergy, seek out a medical professional specializing in food allergies, a nutritionist, or naturopath, who can help you understand and manage your condition. Listed in the resources (page 191) are contacts for finding a professional in your area and obtaining additional information.

The Need for Calcium

It's true that dairy products are a source of calcium. So, when dairy is no longer an option in our diet, we need to find alternative ways to fulfill our daily calcium requirement. Calcium rich foods are plentiful in the plant kingdom, particularly in vegetables, legumes, grains, nuts, seeds, and, yes, even fruit. I was quite surprised to find how many calcium-rich foods I was already eating as part of my normal diet. But the question remained, was I getting enough calcium? To be sure that I would get the calcium my body needed, my doctor recommended that I take a calcium with magnesium supplement, along with vitamin D. She emphasized that I increase the amount of plant-based foods in my diet and that the supplements were simply an insurance policy.

As to which type of calcium supplement works best, Calcium Carbonate or Calcium Citrate both are good. Calcium carbonate is inexpensive but should be taken with an acidic beverage for best utilization. Calcium Citrate is a bit more expensive but is more easily absorbed, particularly for individuals taking any type of acid blockers. Daily calcium requirements vary; check with your doctor to be sure you're at the correct level. When you understand the role calcium plays in your overall health and you know which foods are high in calcium, making an informed decision on how you will meet your daily calcium requirement becomes a lot easier. To find out more, I turned to Kazuko Aoyagi, an expert on the subject of diet, nutrition, and exercise.

Calcium 101 by Kazuko Aoyagi

Most people know that calcium is a mineral necessary for forming and maintaining healthy bones and teeth. However, few people realize that calcium also plays an important role in regulating other body functions, including:

- blood clotting
- blood pressure
- enzyme activation
- contraction and relaxation of muscles (including normal heartbeats)
- nerve transmission
- cell membrane permeability (allowing fluids and other materials to pass in and out of cells)

About 98 percent of the calcium in our body is stored in our bones. When there is not enough calcium present in the diet, calcium is "borrowed" from the bones and released into the bloodstream to maintain these essential body functions. Symptoms of calcium deficiency include osteoporosis, rickets, and impaired muscle contraction (muscle cramps). Over time, dietary calcium deficiency can lead to a loss of bone density, resulting in osteoporosis. However, there is still much debate over whether a lack of dietary calcium is the main cause of loss of bone density. Although dairy foods are often touted as a way to build strong bones, there has never been a study that conclusively links the consumption of dairy products to bone health.

FACTORS CONTRIBUTING TO HEALTHY BONES

Osteoporosis, or the thinning of the bones, is often associated with older people, but the process can start earlier than you might expect. Peak bone mass is achieved by age twenty-five, so it is important to build strong bones as a youth. After age twenty-five, bone mass replenishment slows, and maintaining bone mass becomes increasingly important. Once bones begin to thin, it is hard to reverse the trend with calcium alone. Many factors, such as diet, exercise, medications, hormones, heredity, and lifestyle choices, can influence both the development of bone density and the ability to maintain bone density during the aging process.

Diet. Bones require a wide variety of nutrients to develop normally and to maintain density after maturity. Simply getting the recommended dietary allowance (RDA) of calcium is not enough to keep your bones healthy. Vitamins and minerals, along with proper nutrition, all play a major role. The key nutrients include protein, calcium, phosphorus, magnesium, zinc, boron, manganese, copper, vitamin D, vitamin C, and vitamin K.

Magnesium is especially important, as it is necessary for transporting calcium to the bones. Consuming gallons of milk or taking hundreds of calcium pills will do no good without the presence of magnesium and other elements and minerals. Ironically, drinking too much milk or taking a large dose of calcium supplements can actually cause a calcium imbalance because milk does not contain enough magnesium.

Calcium Absorption. Calcium balance in adults is complex because your body does not absorb all of the calcium you ingest. Once you have met the RDA for calcium of 1,000 milligrams, your body will absorb only what it needs and excrete the rest. Phytates, found in grains, and oxalates, found in green leafy vegetables, reduce the body's ability to absorb calcium somewhat by binding to the calcium so that it cannot be absorbed efficiently. However, recent studies have shown that the amount of fiber, phytates, and oxalates found in the average American diet do not appear to pose a problem for calcium absorption. Research also revealed that vegetarian diets provide adequate amounts of calcium, as measured by body stores.

Exercise. Weight-bearing exercise stimulates bone formation and helps build and maintain strong bones. Thin bones become a major problem when muscles weaken significantly and when bones aren't challenged with weight. A study conducted by NASA showed that weightlessness in space decreased skeletal density in humans and primates by as much as 10 percent. Unfortunately, as we age, most of us become less physically active and the amount of weight-bearing exercise in our daily routine diminishes.

Medications and Hormones. Some medications can actually inhibit the amount of calcium absorbed from food by increasing the calcium lost through the kidneys. One example is a commonly used asthma medication containing corticosteroids. Corticosteroids may also interfere with the production of sex hormones in both men and women, which can contribute to a decrease in bone density. The level of gonadal hormones (estrogen for women and testosterone for men) also appears to regulate bone mass by influencing the absorption of calcium in the intestines. If you are taking medications, you should discuss your nutritional concerns with your doctor.

Heredity and Lifestyle. Lactase deficiency is particularly common among North American African Americans, Asians, Mexicans, Native Americans, and people of Mediterranean or Hispanic origin. In most people, it appears to be an acquired rather than inherited disorder, sometimes beginning after a viral or bacterial infection or other disorder of the gut. Lifestyle choices, such as cigarettes, alcohol, and a high sodium intake and animal proteins can also contribute to calcuim loss. If you're interested in learning more about calcium and nutrition, see the additional resources listed in the bibliography (page 190).

Kazuko Aoyagi, PhD, is an associate director of technology at a pharmaceutical company and an Advanced Study Program Fellow at MIT, where she continues her study in medicine. Dr. Aoyagi writes articles for various publications, including *Prevention* magazine, Impala Racing Team newsletters, and health and fitness websites.

Dairy Alternatives in the Supermarkets

When I started cooking dairy-free, one of my biggest tests of success was cooking for my family and friends. Would they notice a change? Would they find my desserts rich and satisfying? I began in the health food store by going on a shopping spree, loading up with all kinds of alternative products for milk, butter, cheese, and yogurt. If I was going to make dairy-free meals enjoyable, it was important to find alternatives I liked. I tried cooking and baking with some of these products and soon found out that not all dairy alternatives are created equal. I also realized that I couldn't run to the natural food store every time I needed something. So I changed my approach: I began looking very closely at the new products making their way into supermarkets and was pleasantly surprised to find almost all of the alternatives I was seeking.

Recognizing how busy our lives are these days, I've made sure that all of the recipes in this cookbook use ingredients that can be purchased from your neighborhood supermarket. *The Dairy-Free & Gluten-Free Kitchen* uses common, easily obtained ingredients. If you have difficulty finding a product used here, turn to the manufacturers and distributors section in the resources (page 192) for a comprehensive guide with contact information that will allow you to communicate with the manufacturer directly.

FOOD LABELING

The labeling used on food products is a very useful tool when you are trying to eliminate dairy products from your diet completely. But like everything else, ingredient labels can change without notice. It's a good idea to read the label every time you purchase a product. Manufacturers are always making changes to products for a wide variety of reasons, or they may elect to drop a product from their line altogether. It is best not to assume that a product or brand you've bought before will be the same the next time you buy it. If you have a question about a specific product, contact the manufacturer (see page 192).

When reading a label, you need to know the dairy buzzwords. Take time to learn the ones you don't know, write them down, and carry the list with you for reference when shopping. Dairy and its derivatives can be found in the most unusual places, including packaged lunch meats, some of which contain sodium caseinate, casein, whey, or nonfat dry milk; some brands of margarine, sliced bread, mayonnaise, semi-sweet chocolate, and potato chips. The most surprising items I've come across containing dairy derivatives are cosmetics, vitamins, and medicines both over the counter and prescription. If you find any of the following terms listed on a package label, the product contains dairy.

TERMS ON DAIRY LABELS

1 percent milk

2 percent milk

a2 milk™

acidophilus milk

artificial butter flavor

butter

butter fat

butter oil

buttermilk

casein

caseinates in any form (calcium, potassium, sodium, magnesium, and ammonium)

cheese

condensed milk

cottage cheese

cream

cream cheese

curds

custard

dry milk

evaporated milk

feta cheese

ghee

goat milk

half-and-half

hydrolysates

ice cream

ice milk

kefir

lactalbumin

lactoglobulin

lactose

lactose-free milks

lactulose

low-fat milk

malted milk

margarine (some brands)

milk proteins

milk solids

milkfat

nonfat milk

nougat

pasteurized cheese

pudding

rennet casein

sheep milk

sherbet

skim milk

sour cream

whey

whole milk

yogurt

With growing public awareness of the issue of lactose intolerance, manufacturers are recognizing a new market segment and are beginning to respond to the demand for lactose-free products.

If you are strictly lactose intolerant, this is good news. However, if you have a dairy allergy, lactose-free products won't help and should be avoided. A product label might indicate that it is lactose free or that it is a dairy alternative, leading you to believe that the product does not contain dairy. It still might contain milk proteins, however, which can trigger allergic reactions. Good examples of products labeled nondairy that contain dairy proteins include some brands of coffee creamers, cheese alternatives, and nondairy whipped toppings.

KOSHER SYMBOLS

Special codes or symbols located on the front of a package label can also help identify products that contain dairy. These symbols are actually kosher markings that comply with Jewish dietary laws. The FDA does not regulate these symbols and it is not mandatory that they appear on food labels. However, when they do appear, they can helpful. "D" indicates that the product contains dairy. Note that sometimes a label will list a D yet the ingredients list will not indicate the presence of milk.

This can occur for two reasons: The product contains natural flavorings from dairy ingredients; or the equipment was previously used with dairy products that could have left residual amounts, making it unsafe for people with dairy allergies. (I found an example of double-duty equipment use when I was purchasing a bag of tortilla chips and noticed that the package had a D listed on it. The ingredients clearly stated that no dairy was present, so I called the manufacturer. They explained to me that the equipment had previously been used to produce chips containing dairy, and so they used the D label as a precaution for possible cross contamination.)

"DE" stands for dairy equipment. This means that the product was produced using equipment that was also used to manufacture products containing dairy. The DE symbol is not being used as often because D covers a broader range of possibilities.

"Pareve" or "Parve" indicates that the product does not contain either meat or dairy, it is casein free. "K," "U," and "OU" indicate that the product has been manufactured in compliance with Jewish dietary standards and laws. These three symbols have nothing to do with whether or not a dairy ingredient has been used in the product.

MILK ALTERNATIVES

When I began my dairy-free diet twenty years ago, finding milk alternatives in the supermarket was difficult at best. However, in today's markets, you'd be hard-pressed not to find any number of soy milk or nondairy beverages to choose from. Manufacturers are offering a wide selection of satisfying milk alternatives by using rice, soy, almond, hazelnut, hemp, coconut, millet, and potatoes. To add to the choices, these nondairy beverages come in plain (also called original or unsweetened) as well as in an array of flavors, such as vanilla, chocolate, carob, and seasonal offerings. Additionally, nondairy beverages are offered in a range of fat contents, as organic or not, and many are enriched with calcium and vitamins. The benefit of the enriched varieties is that they provide as much calcium and vitamins A and D as dairy milk. With so many options, your dairy-free milk choice comes down to personal preference and taste.

When cooking savory recipes, my preference is an unsweetened organic nondairy almond beverage, as I have found that even the plain beverage alternatives can impart a sweetness that's often not suitable for most savory dishes. However, for desserts or any of the bread recipes, any unsweetened or sweetened nondairy beverage will work just fine.

The recipes in this cookbook were developed using unsweetened organic soy milk, almond, hemp, or rice nondairy beverage, which all work equally well. Do not use any of the flavored milks unless the recipe calls for it. Whether you choose a shelf-stable or refrigerated nondairy milk, each time you use it, be sure to shake the container. It's normal for the milk to separate when it settles. If you are on a gluten-free diet check that your choice of milk alternative is in fact gluten-free. Some nondairy beverages use barley malt as a sweetener or grains, such as oats, making them unsafe for people with gluten intolerance.

Shelf-stable nondairy milk substitutes have the benefit of convenience. I often buy a case at a time, because the vacuum-sealed aseptic packaging allows the product to be kept unopened in the pantry for several months. If you check the date stamped on the package and monitor your supply, you will always have milk on hand. Once the container is opened, it will stay fresh for seven to ten days in the refrigerator, just as milk will.

BUTTER ALTERNATIVES

To eliminate unnecessary fats, I have greatly reduced the amount of recipes requiring margarine in this book. However, for the few that do use margarine, the best I have found for all around use is Earth Balance® natural buttery spread. This spread can be used in any recipe calling for butter and in the same amounts. In addition to being dairy-free it is also gluten-free, vegan, non-GMO, and free of hydrogenated oils, trans fats, and artificial ingredients. And for those who have a soy intolerance, they also offer a soy-free version. In baked goods I've minimized the fat by using fat replacers, such as mashed bananas, pureed prunes, applesauce, silken tofu, or soy yogurt.

Other margarines are available in the market, many still made with harmful hydrogenated oils, trans fats, artificial color, flavors, and preservatives. It's important to note that just because a product is called "margarine" does not mean it is dairy-free. Many margarines contain milk proteins, whey, or buttermilk used as flavor enhancers, so it's important to look for the word *pareve* or *vegan* on the packaging.

EGGS

A common mistake is considering eggs a dairy product. Although they are often found in the dairy section of supermarkets, eggs are not a dairy product. For the best flavor and nutritional value, look for organic cage-free eggs from free-range or pasture-raised hens. For those who follow a vegan diet or have an egg protein allergy, all of the recipes note if they contain eggs. Although eggs are used in several of the bread recipes, you can use an egg replacer; however, the results will produce a slightly denser outcome. For prepared egg replacer product information, turn to the manufacturers and distributors section in the resources (page 192). For recipes requiring two or less eggs you can elect one of the following substitutions:

Silken tofu: For quick breads, cakes, and custards, 2 tablespoons equals 1 egg.

For quick breads, yeasted breads, and cakes: 1 tablespoon finely ground flaxseed (meal) whisked with 3 tablespoons water makes $1/4$ cup, which equals 2 eggs in a recipe.

YOGURT

There are several very tasty dairy-free yogurts available, all offering the probiotic benefits of a dairy-based yogurt for enhanced intestinal health. Look for dairy-free yogurts made from soy, almond, rice, or coconut milk; most are gluten-free. Or you can make your own dairy-free yogurt by following the Nut Milk Yogurt recipe on page 174.

SOUR CREAM

Several sour cream alternatives are available, but be careful as many contain casein, a milk protein. Instead, make your own with the Lean Sour Cream recipe (page 125). It is a fantastic sour cream substitute and can be used in Beef Stroganoff (page 92) or atop a baked potato.

CHEESE

Over the years in the food business, the number one complaint I've heard from the public is not being able to eat cheese. Well, manufacturers are listening and have created many new cheese alternatives. They can be made from soy, rice, almonds, or tapioca and are available in stores or online. Most cheese alternatives are fine to use if you are lactose intolerant and can handle milk proteins. However, if you have a dairy allergy, you'll need to carefully examine the ingredients label as many do contain the milk protein casein, which is added so the cheese will melt. Or look for the word *vegan*, which ensures that the cheese is free of all animal products. Please note that if you are on a gluten-free diet, check the label, as some cheese alternatives may contain gluten ingredients.

Cheese alternatives are an acquired taste, so be prepared to try several different brands and flavors before you find one you like. Personally I prefer making my own cheese, and after you try some of the recipes in this book—Creamy Macadamia Pine Nut Cheese (page 175), Cheesy Mac 'n' Nut Cheese (page 103), and Mushroom Kale Lasagna (page 94)—I bet you won't even miss the dairy cheese.

ICE CREAM

Sorbet is widely available in many supermarkets and comes in several different brands and flavors, including chocolate, lemon, raspberry, and assorted tropical flavors. Natural food stores are still the best bet for a good selection of soy, rice, coconut, hemp, or almond-based frozen desserts. Some flavors may contain gluten ingredients so be sure to check the label.

TOFU

Also known as bean curd, tofu can usually be found in your supermarket's produce section, although some stores have a special meat/dairy alternative section for it. Tofu is produced in silken, soft, medium, firm, and extra-firm textures and in low-fat calcium-enriched, organic, and sprouted varieties.

The most common variety, "cotton"-style tofu, is primarily sold packed in liquid in plastic tubs and must be kept refrigerated. Silken-style tofu is often packaged in aseptic boxes, has a silky-smooth appearance and texture, and does not need refrigeration until it is opened. Silken or soft-pressed tofu is best used in smoothies, sauces, dressings, and other recipes that are blended. Medium and firm tofu work best crumbled in casseroles and for cheesecake. The firm and extra-firm types are best suited for stir-fries, grilling, soups, and salads.

Once you have opened a container of tofu, store any that you have left over by immersing it in water in a container with a tight-fitting lid and keep it in the refrigerator. Change the water daily, and the tofu will keep for about five days.

TEMPEH

Tempeh is fermented soybeans pressed to form a cake and is commonly sold alongside tofu in the refrigerated section. Some flavors may contain gluten ingredients so be sure to check the label. Tempeh is an excellent protein source and can be used in a recipe to substitute ground meat. This versatile plant protein can be crumbled, sliced or cubed, grilled, sautéed, steamed, or stir-fried.

Understanding Gluten

For millions of Americans, wheat and gluten can contribute to or cause serious health problems. In the United States, 1 in every 133 people has celiac disease, a genetic intolerance to gluten affecting the lining of the small intestine. Beyond celiac disease, an estimated 17 to 21 million are non-celiac gluten sensitive, while another 3 million have a true wheat allergy. Just as in the case of dairy, wheat and gluten are prevalent in the foods we eat everyday. Apart from the better-known culprits, such as bread, pasta, and pizza, gluten can be found in the most unexpected places. This section will serve as an overview for anyone who suspects they may have a problem with gluten. Additional gluten-free information sources and lab testing resources can be obtained in the bibliography and the resources (see page 190).

What Is Gluten?

Gluten is the general term used for proteins that are found in specific cereal grains. Think of it as glue; it is the sticky, stretchy protein that forms when wheat flour is mixed with water; it is what holds baked goods together and gives them their spring. Gluten is found in all varieties of wheat, (durum, semolina, faro, kamut, einkorn, graham, and spelt) along with rye, barley, and triticale (a mixture of wheat and rye). A special note about oats: Although oats do not inherently contain gluten they are often processed with the same milling equipment and stored in the same grain silos as wheat. As a result, gluten cross contamination occurs making oats unstable for individuals on a gluten-free, wheat-free diet. However, there is good news! Certified gluten-free oats are now available in the market and online; see the manufacturers and distributors section in the resources (page 192).

Celiac Disease

Celiac disease, also referred to as celic sprue or gluten sensitive enteropathy (and called coeliac outside the United States) is a genetic autoimmune disorder that causes damage to the small hairs called *villi* that line the small intestine. Under a microscope, the villi look like small finger-like projections lining the small intestine and play a critical role in the digestion of food and assimilation of nutrients. When individuals with celiac disease ingest gluten containing grains and/or their byproducts, specific antibodies are triggered that begin to wear down and damage the villi. Here's a visual I like to use. A healthy intestinal lining looks a bit like a shaggy carpet with all of the fibers moving in harmony, sweeping food along and producing enzymes to aid in proper digestion. Over time, the intestinal lining of an individual with celiac disease looks like a worn, flattened shag carpet. Now, instead of the nutrients pausing for assimilation, they instead pass quickly through the gut, leading to a host of malabsorption issues.

Celiac disease is very often misdiagnosed because it can present itself in many different ways, including but not limited to: gastrointestinal distress, such as IBS-like symptoms; chronic or intermittent diarrhea, constipation, bloating, or cramps. Yet other individuals may not manifest any gastrointestinal upset, but instead experience brain fog, fatigue, weight loss, anemia, depression, migraines, asthma, irritability, infertility, or a host of skin conditions, such as a blistery rash called *dermatitis herpetiformis*. Once considered an obscure malady, taking years to diagnose, celiac disease is now getting mainstream attention. As a result, diagnosis is becoming much quicker through the use of blood tests, genetic testing, and small bowel biopsy.

Lactose Intolerance and Celiac Disease

As discussed earlier, lactose intolerance is related to the body's inability to produce the enzyme lactase, which is needed to digest lactose (milk sugar). Because celiac disease damages the villi where the lactase enzyme is manufactured, it is very common for newly diagnosed celiac patients to experience temporary lactose intolerance. For some celiac individuals who are not predisposed to lactose intolerance, when a gluten-free diet is adopted, the villi will begin to recover and lactase enzyme production will resume, enabling the individual to once again tolerate dairy. This healing process can take up to a year. However, some individuals predisposed to lactose intolerance or a dairy sensitivity may conclude that dairy is no longer an option for them.

It is very important to note that if you suspect that you might be a candidate for celiac disease, get tested first with a medical professional before you embark on a gluten-free diet. If you eliminate gluten and then get tested, the blood panel may come back with a false negative result, leaving you to always wonder. Currently the only medical treatment for individuals with celiac disease is the complete elimination of all traces of gluten from the diet. Once on a gluten-free diet, some people begin to feel better almost immediately whereas others can take up to a year or more. The good news is that with lifelong adherence to a gluten-free diet your intestinal villi will fully heal, allowing you to absorb the nutrients you need to be healthy.

Gluten Sensitivity

Unlike celiac disease, there are no clinical tests that will diagnose if an individual has a gluten sensitivity. Non-celiac gluten sensitivity shares many of the same symptoms as celiac disease and thus is often confused for the disease. What sets gluten sensitivity apart from celiac disease is that it does not cause any measurable intestinal villi damage. As with a dairy sensitivity, gluten-sensitive individuals can experience immediate or systemic delayed reactions that develop over several days and may become chronic. Symptoms include, but are not limited to, gastrointestinal discomfort, such as diarrhea, bloating to constipation, flatulence (gas), leaky gut, brain fog, joint pain, tingling fingers, headaches, chronic fatigue, infertility, depression, ADHD, or autistic behaviors.

Wheat Allergy

A wheat allergy (an IgE mediated allergy) triggers a completely different bodily function than does celiac disease or gluten sensitivity. Unlike gluten sensitivity, clinical blood tests are available to test for a wheat allergy. These same tests can also determine if you have other protein allergies to dairy, eggs, tree nuts, peanuts, fish, shellfish, and soy. As with a dairy allergy, individuals with a wheat allergy can experience an immediate anaphylactic allergic reaction or delayed reactions, such as hives, respiratory problems, headaches, and stomach discomfort. With a wheat allergy, individuals may tolerate rye, barley, and oats but must avoid wheat in all its forms.

Gluten-Free Alternatives in the Supermarket

For years now I have worked with individuals and families challenged with special dietary needs to make the transition to a gluten-free and dairy-free lifestyle. One key component is navigating the supermarket maze and learning about the ever-increasing alternative products emerging on grocery shelves. However, there is a caveat with many of these product alternatives: They are not necessarily healthier options. Sure, they may be safe from a food intolerance, sensitivity, allergy perspective; however, from a nutritional perspective they are often loaded with added sweeteners, fats, and are low in fiber, all traits typical of processed foods. For optimal nutrition, choose fresh, whole foods and when you do purchase processed products, read the ingredients and nutritional facts so that you can make an informed, healthful decision.

FOOD LABELING

If you are newly diagnosed with celiac disease, gluten sensitivity, or a wheat allergy, it is vital that you become an expert label reader and familiarize yourself with the foods you can eat. Like dairy, gluten is a ubiquitous ingredient in a multitude of products, including ones that may surprise you. The following list is divided into items that definitely have gluten and those that require a label-read.

FINDING GLUTEN ON LABELS

All of the products below will contain gluten, unless they have been specially formulated to be gluten-free. For example, some lunch meats have a glaze that contains gluten, but not all—they are brand specific. Oats do not naturally contain gluten, but oats processed in the United States do because of cross contamination, unless they are certified as gluten-free oats. On the other hand, oats grown and packaged in Scotland and Ireland typically are gluten-free. However, *Scottish oats*, a name that is used loosely for the style of oat, does not guarantee that the oats are truly from Scotland. There are now gluten-free beers available, as well as pastas. The nuances can be confusing, so for greater precision in identification, the first list presents products that definitely contain gluten, while the second list notes products that more often than not contain gluten, while allowing that there are gluten-free alternatives available. Both lists are intended to be a quick reference for identifying problem, or potentially problematic, foods.

Stop! Contains Gluten

additives, such as: dextrin, hydrolyzed vegetable protein, starches, caramel color

barley

barley malt

barley starch

breading and coating mixes

bullion cubes

communion wafers

couscous

croutons

cracked wheat

flour

malt

matzo meal

natural or artificial flavoring or coloring

panko

rye

soy sauce

sprouted wheat

tabouli

wheat (durum, semolina, faro, kamut, einkorn, graham, spelt)

wheat bran

wheat germ

wheat germ oil

wheat meal

wheat stabilizers

wheat starch

white flour

whole wheat

Caution! May Contain Gluten

- baking power
- beer
- brown rice syrup
- corn tortillas
- dressings
- energy bars
- imitation seafood
- licorice and candy
- lipstick and lip gloss
- lunch meats
- marinades
- mustard powder
- oat bran or germ
- oatmeal
- over the counter medications
- pasta
- prescription drugs
- seasoning mixes
- soups and broths
- vitamin mineral supplements

READING A LABEL

The Food Allergen Labeling and Consumer Protection act (FALCPA) ensures that clear labeling of the top eight allergens (milk, wheat, eggs, tree nuts, peanuts, fish, shellfish, and soy) appear on all product labels. Beyond that, some manufacturers have voluntarily sought third-party gluten-free certification from one of the following organizations: Celiac Sprue Association (CSA), National Foundation for Celiac Awareness (NFCA), or the Gluten Intolerance Group (GIG), also known as the Gluten-Free Certification Organization (GFOC). To be sure the product you choose is gluten-free look for the certificating organization's symbol.

ALTERNATIVE FLOURS

No wheat, no worries, you can still make your favorite foods. In fact, gluten-free alternative grains and flours provide a world of delicious possibilities. The following gluten-free grains, nuts, seeds, roots, legumes, and milled flours are all naturally gluten-free [the (*) denotes recommended refrigeration]:

- amaranth*
- arrowroot, flour or starch
- brown rice*
- buckwheat*
- corn
- garbanzo (chickpea)*
- garfava*
- guar gum*
- millet*
- nut meal flours* (almond, hazelnut, coconut)
- certified gluten-free oats, if tolerated
- potato
- quinoa*
- seeds*: chia, flax, hemp
- sorghum*
- soy*
- tapioca, flour or starch
- teff*
- white rice
- xanthan gum*

Alternative flours can be expensive and are often used in small quantities. To protect your investment from going rancid, store any unused portions in an airtight container in the refrigerator or freezer.

Gluten-free flours each have their own characteristics and must be combined in a recipe to achieve consistent results. After working with

the **dairy-free** and **gluten-free** kitchen

all of these flours in various proportions, I have developed what I consider an excellent master gluten-free flour mix (page 172). I start with rice flour, preferably brown rice for added nutrition. Next comes potato starch and tapioca or arrowroot flours for their lightness and browning capabilities. Lastly, a protein flour is added for both nutrition and structure; my preference is sorghum flour for its neutral flavor. This mix is ideal for multi purpose use whether you're creating a savory or sweet dish. Occasionally recipes will have an additional flour added, and the reason for this is to change the flavor profile, as in the Almond Biscotti (page 167).

Xanthan and guar gum: These binding agents lend elasticity to baked goods. If a recipe requires either, it will be called for in the ingredients, but please note that a little goes a long way—use too much and the dish will be gummy; use too little and it will crumble too easily.

Organic Products in the Supermarket

Responding to consumer demand, many supermarkets now carry certified organic produce, meats, poultry, eggs, and grocery items. Sometimes these items may cost a little more, but they are well worth it for several reasons:

Any chance to reduce our exposure to long-lasting pesticide, herbicide, and fungicide residue, genetically modified organisms (GMO), irradiation, sewage sludge, artificial growth hormones, synthetic preservatives, and antibiotics in our food is always beneficial.

Purchasing these products will let the store know that organic products are important to you and your family. Supermarkets are more likely to expand their selection of these products when they see an increased demand. It encourages

farmers to preserve the environment by utilizing alternative farming methods that involve enriching the soil through composting, crop rotation, cover crops, and natural pest control.

Organic livestock standards ensure that animals are not administered synthetic growth hormones, they are fed organic feed, and live in species-appropriate natural living conditions.

Organic farming conserves our natural resources, promotes better health, supports sustainable agricultural practice, and creates a safer working environment for farm workers. Organic standards cover all aspects of organic livestock, crop production, organic certification, processing, and marketing. Products that meet the organic standards display an official United States Department of Agriculture (USDA) organic seal, making it easier for consumers to identify certified organic products.

About the Recipes

Food is a delight for the senses. As you prepare these recipes, observe how the herbs and spices interact with each other and how the flavors blend. Throughout the book you will find recipes with the instructions, "Taste and correct the seasonings." As a general rule, your seasonings should complement the dish, not overpower it. If you can taste one seasoning as a separate element, you may have used too much. Start with a small amount and build from there. Be patient. You can always add more salt or pepper, tarragon, or vinegar, but you can't undo it once you've added it. It's important to note that many seasonings intensify as they simmer, so take it slow and enjoy the rich aromas as you go.

Whenever possible, I have prepared all of the recipes in this book using organic, seasonal, and local ingredients. Whether they are from our neighborhood market, the local farmers' market, or my backyard organic garden, I believe organics are more nutritious and simply taste better than their conventional counterparts. Many of the recipes use some basic organic pantry ingredients including organic dried fruits, nuts, and seeds. I recommend that you keep these ingredients on-hand as they are used in many of the recipes. Store the fruit in airtight containers in your panty, and the nuts and seeds in the freezer; they will stay fresh longer.

You'll notice that many of the recipes provide you with an option to cook without the use of extracted cooking oils. I've done this because reducing and removing unnecessary oils from the recipes eliminates a substantial amount of excess fat and calories from our daily diet. For recipes that do use oil, I recommend using only expeller-pressed or cold-pressed oils; both utilize chemical-free pressing methods. I am not advocating a fat-free diet; we need fat, but good fat from whole foods, such as seeds, nuts, olives, and avocados, are the fats we want to emphasize. I've identified the recipes in this book that are oil-free, and in many of the savory recipes you can simply substitute the oil you might normally use with an equal amount of water, vegetable stock, or chicken stock.

So how do we cook without oil? We'll use a method called steam-sauté that works like this: Start with a hot pan, add your vegetables according to the recipe directions, and stir frenquently.

Keeping the vegetables moving will keep them from sticking to the bottom of the pan. You'll notice the natural sugars in the vegetables will begin to caramelize, giving them a sweet, intense flavor. Next, you'll want to steam for texture. Simply add 2 tablespoons of liquid, typically water, stock, or wine in small amounts to deglaze the pan, then proceed with the recipe.

In addition to the reduction of oil in the recipes, I've also reduced the amount of refined sugar, whenever possible, by substituting it with a delicious, whole-food, fiber-rich sweetener called Date Syrup (page 189). In less than five minutes you can blend up a batch, ensuring you'll always have a nutritious sweetner on hand. If dates are unavailable, then honey can be substituted, but using honey will change the nutritional benefits and flavor profile of the recipe.

My goal is to help you learn about the wonderful alternatives to dairy and gluten—for yourself or for family members and friends. In the pages that follow, you'll find a collection of recipes that will give you the tools to choose healthier options while still offering the occasional decadent treat. None of the recipes contain wheat, gluten, or dairy in any form, including lactose, casein, or milk proteins. However, they are loaded with flavor, creatively conceived, and delicious. I hope that preparing the recipes in the pages that follow will be a true adventure and will add much to your enjoyment of healthful, dairy-free, and gluten-free living. Now, let's get started.

Bon appétit and *prijatino*!

breakfast

Breakfast foods needn't be limited to the morning; they can be eaten anytime, day or night. I've included recipes for an assortment of breakfast treats—from quick grab-and-go nutrient-packed bars, smoothies, and comforting grains to traditional favorites like pancakes and French toast—all of which typically use dairy and wheat. Try any of these dairy- and gluten-free recipes as a quick bite, a leisurely brunch, hors d'oeuvres, or a gratifying supper. Whatever your pleasure, these breakfasts hold no boundaries and are positively delicious.

basic smoothie recipe

SERVES 1 TO 2

Quick and nourishing smoothies offer a great way to start the day or a quick pick-me-up after a workout. Adding chia or flax seeds gives an extra boost of nutrition by providing omega-3s, fiber, and protein. Or turn your smoothie into a green powerhouse by adding $1/2$ cup of frozen greens, such as kale, collards, or spinach to the mix, or add a teaspoon of either spirulina or chlorella powder. If you prefer a sweeter tasting smoothie but without the added sugar, add 4 to 5 drops of liquid stevia to the mix or a pitted date.

Combine all of the ingredients in a blender, cover, and whirl at top speed for approximately 1 minute or until smooth. Pour into a glass, garnish with a straw, and enjoy. When making fruit smoothies, adding ice to the blender is a matter of personal choice; if you are using frozen fruit in place of fresh fruit you may elect to omit the ice.

blueberry banana smoothie

Free of EGG SOY SUGAR OIL

1 ripe banana, cut into 2-inch chunks

1 cup fresh blueberries (or berry of choice)

1 cup cold water

$3/4$ cup Dairy Milk Alternative (page 173)

1 tablespoon raw almond butter

1 tablespoon chia (saba) or flax seeds

Blend as instructed in the Basic Smoothie Recipe.

tropical smoothie

Free of EGG SOY* SUGAR OIL

1 cup cubed pineapple

1 cup sliced fresh mango

³/₄ cup or 1 (6-ounce) container plain dairy-free yogurt*

1 cup coconut milk beverage, coconut water, or Dairy Milk Alternative (page 173)

1 cup cold water

1 tablespoon chia (saba) or flax seeds

Blend as instructed in the Basic Smoothie Recipe.

spicy green smoothie

Free of EGG SOY NUT SUGAR OIL

¹/₂ pound vine ripened tomato, cored, cut into quarters

1 cup cold water

1 cup tightly packed fresh spinach

¹/₂ ripe avocado, peeled and pitted

1 jalapeño pepper, seeded

2 green onions, white and green parts

¹/₄ bunch cilantro or parsley

1 tablespoon freshly squeezed lime juice (about 1 lime)

Dash gluten-free hot sauce, or to taste

Blend as instructed in the Basic Smoothie Recipe.

breakfast seed *and* fruit bars

Free of EGG SOY NUT SUGAR OIL

MAKES 10 BARS

These tasty bars are simple to assemble and ideal for breakfast on the go. They contain no refined sugar, provide a healthy dose of fiber, and are chock-full of protein. To change up the recipe, substitute your favorite dried fruit or any combination of chopped nuts.

1 cup apple juice

6 medjool dates, pitted

4 prunes, pitted

1 teaspoon gluten-free vanilla extract

³/₄ cup gluten-free rolled oats or quinoa flakes

¹/₂ cup Gluten-Free Flour Mix (page 172)

¹/₂ teaspoon cinnamon

¹/₄ teaspoon salt

³/₄ cup raw pumpkin seeds

³/₄ cup raw sunflower seeds

¹/₂ cup dried cranberries or raisins

Preheat the oven to 350°F. Cut a piece of parchment paper to fit an 8 by 8 by 2-inch baking dish. Lightly spray the dish with cooking spray and arrange the parchment paper on the bottom of the dish, set aside.

TO PREPARE THE BARS: Place the apple juice, dates, prunes, and vanilla in a blender. Set aside. Meanwhile, in a large bowl combine the oats, flour, cinnamon, and salt. Mix together with a large spoon until blended. Add the pumpkin seeds, sunflower seeds, and cranberries, stirring to incorporate.

Cover the blender and pulse the date mixture 5 or 6 times to break up the fruit. Whirl at top speed for approximately 30 seconds or until the mixture is just blended. Pour the date mixture into the flour mixture, stirring until incorporated.

TO BAKE THE BARS: Transfer the dough to the prepared baking dish. Using your hands or the back of a spatula, very firmly press the mixture into the pan. Bake until lightly browned, about 20 minutes. Allow the mixture to cool completely in the pan, about 1 hour. Turn the mixture out onto a cutting board, remove the parchment paper, and slice into 10 (1¹/₂ by 4-inch) bars. To store the bars, wrap each piece in plastic wrap and transfer to an airtight container for up to 3 days or freeze for longer storage.

nutty berry muesli

Free of EGG SOY* SUGAR OIL

MAKES 5 CUPS

This nutrient-packed breakfast cereal can be eaten either cold or hot, but either way it's delicious. There really is no right or wrong way to make muesli; it's an amazingly versatile cereal, so get creative and have fun. This recipe will get you started, but play around with any combination of dried or fresh fruit, coconut, raw nuts, and seeds. I've made this version with organic raw nuts and seeds, and unsulfured dried fruit.

2 cups gluten-free rolled oats

1 cup quinoa flakes

$^3/_4$ cup dried cranberries

$^1/_2$ cup chopped dried apricots

$^1/_4$ cup slivered almonds

$^1/_4$ cup chopped walnuts

$^1/_4$ cup ground flax meal or chia (saba) seed

Dairy Milk Alternative (page 173)

Plain dairy-free yogurt*

TO PREPARE THE CEREAL: Combine the oats, quinoa, cranberries, apricots, almonds, and walnuts in a large bowl, and mix to blend. Store any unused cereal in a container with a tight-fitting lid, and refrigerate.

TO PREPARE 2 SERVINGS OF COLD MUESLI: Place $^1/_2$ cup of cereal in a bowl with 1 cup of yogurt or milk; stir to blend. Let stand for 15 minutes or place in a covered container in the refrigerator overnight. Sprinkle with flax meal before serving. Serve with additional milk if desired.

TO PREPARE 2 SERVINGS OF HOT MUESLI: Combine 1 cup of cereal with 1 cup of water or milk in a saucepan over medium-high heat. Bring the mixture to a boil. Decrease the heat to low and cook for 3 to 5 minutes, stirring occasionally. Ladle into bowls and sprinkle with flax meal. Serve with additional milk if desired.

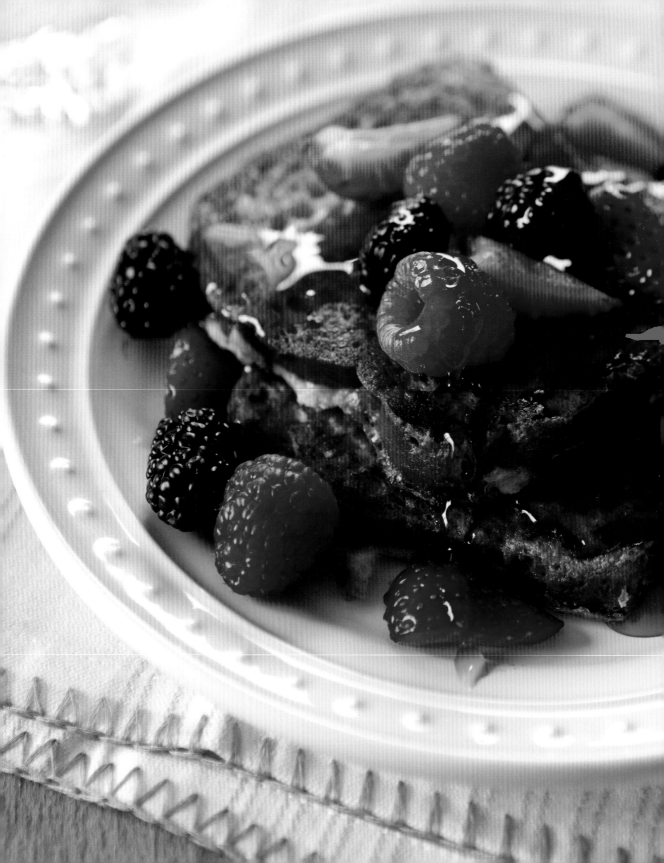

classic french toast

Free of SOY NUT* OIL

SERVES 4

The smell of French toast always gets my family out of bed in a hurry. The combination of sweet maple syrup with crispy, yet soft bread makes for a wonderful taste sensation. Any type of gluten-free bread can be used here. Serve with pure maple syrup and top with sliced fresh fruit.

4 large eggs

1¼ cups Dairy Milk Alternative (page 173)

12 slices day-old Fiber-Rich Sandwich Bread, sliced ½ inch thick (page 137)

2 tablespoons coconut * or canola oil, for greasing the griddle

Pure maple syrup, warmed

2 cups sliced seasonal fresh fruit (banana, mango, berries, peaches)

TO PREPARE THE EGG AND BREAD: Whisk together the eggs and milk in a bowl until well blended. Pour the egg mixture into an 8 by 11 by 2-inch baking dish or a shallow bowl. Soak the bread in the egg mixture, turning carefully to coat and saturate, for 2 to 3 minutes.

TO MAKE THE FRENCH TOAST: Preheat a griddle or heavy skillet over medium-high heat (375°F for an electric griddle). Lightly grease the griddle with oil. Transfer the egg-soaked bread to the hot griddle. Cook until lightly browned, about 3 minutes. Using a spatula, carefully flip the bread and continue cooking until lightly browned, 3 to 4 minutes longer. Serve immediately.

buckwheat pancakes *with* seasonal fruit

Free of EGG SOY NUT OIL

SERVES 4

However you like your pancakes—thick or thin— these are sure to please. My mom would make pancakes by the dozen, as the five of us kids vied to see who could eat the most. (One of my brothers would always win.) Today, we still make these all-time favorites, and thanks to Marc and Maureen Kellond, two amazing vegan chefs who shared their favorite pancake recipe with me, they're healthier too. If you like your pancakes thicker, use a little less milk. If thinner pancakes are your pleasure, use up to 1/4 cup more.

1 tablespoon ground flaxseed

3 tablespoons water

1 tablespoon pure maple syrup

1 teaspoon apple cider vinegar

1½ cups Gluten-Free Flour Mix (page 172)

½ cup buckwheat flour

½ teaspoon gluten-free baking powder

½ teaspoon baking soda

¼ teaspoon cinnamon

¼ teaspoon xanthan gum

¼ teaspoon salt

2 cups Dairy Milk Alternative (page 173)

Canola or coconut oil, for greasing the griddle

Pure maple syrup, warmed

2 cups sliced seasonal fresh fruit and berries

TO PREPARE THE BATTER: Combine the flax, water, maple syrup, and vinegar in a bowl and whisk to blend. Set aside. In a separate large bowl, combine the flour, buckwheat flour, baking powder, baking soda, cinnamon, xanthan gum, and salt and mix together with a whisk. Whisk the flax mixture for 1 minute until slightly thickened, and add the milk, whisking to blend. Pour the milk mixture into the flour mixture and whisk until the batter is smooth.

TO MAKE THE PANCAKES: Preheat a griddle or heavy skillet over medium-high heat (375°F on an electric griddle). Lightly grease the griddle with oil. Ladle enough batter onto the hot griddle to make a 6-inch-diameter pancake. Cook until bubbles cover the pancake's surface, 2 to 3 minutes, then flip the pancake using a spatula. Continue to cook the pancake for 2 to 3 minutes longer, or until golden brown. Do not press on the pancake after flipping. Continue making pancakes with the remaining batter. Serve immediately with warm maple syrup, and top with sliced fruit and berries.

potato pancakes

MAKES TWELVE 4-INCH PANCAKES

Golden brown and crisp on the outside, moist and tender on the inside, these delicious griddle cakes are surprisingly simple to make. Use high-quality oil to fry the pancakes, making sure it is very hot before you add the batter. This will ensure light, crispy pancakes every time. Have them for breakfast or alongside the main course for dinner, but definitely serve them with applesauce.

2 pounds russet potatoes

1/4 cup Gluten-Free Flour Mix (page 172)

1 teaspoon gluten-free baking powder

1 teaspoon salt

1/4 teaspoon freshly ground black pepper

2 large eggs, beaten

4 green onions, white and green parts, thinly sliced

1/4 cup canola oil, more if needed

3 cups Applesauce (page 134) or 1 (24-ounce) jar applesauce

TO PREPARE THE POTATOES: Line a dinner plate with a double layer of cheesecloth. Peel the potatoes and then, using the largest holes on a grater, grate them onto the cheesecloth. Gather up the corners of the cheesecloth and squeeze the potatoes to extract any liquid.

TO PREPARE THE BATTER: In a large bowl, whisk together the flour, baking powder, salt, and pepper. Add the eggs, green onions, and potatoes, and stir to blend.

TO MAKE THE PANCAKES: Line a plate with several layers of paper towel and set aside. Heat 2 tablespoons of the oil in a cast-iron skillet or heavy nonstick skillet over medium-high heat. Spoon the batter by 1/4 cupfuls onto the hot skillet, flattening them slightly with the back of the spoon. Fry until their undersides are golden brown, 3 to 5 minutes. Flip the pancakes over and cook 3 to 4 minutes longer. Transfer the pancakes to the prepared plate. Continue cooking the pancakes, adding oil as needed, 2 tablespoons at a time, with the remaining batter. Serve hot with applesauce.

crab *and* artichoke frittata

Free of SOY   NUT   SUGAR

SERVES 4 TO 6

The colors and flavors of this frittata are deliciously appealing, making it a Mother's Day brunch favorite at our house. Frittatas are incredibly versatile and easy to prepare; take one on your next picnic, or try serving it as a light supper with a salad of vine-ripened tomatoes and whole basil leaves drizzled with extra virgin olive oil, balsamic vinegar, and a turn or two of coarse salt and cracked pepper. Sliced into bite-size pieces and served at room temperature, frittatas also make an attractive yet simple appetizer.

10 large eggs

$^1/_2$ cup Dairy Milk Alternative (page 173)

$^3/_4$ teaspoon salt

$^1/_4$ teaspoon freshly ground black pepper

2 red bell peppers, roasted (see page 182) and chopped

1 cup stemmed, chopped fresh spinach, tightly packed (about $^1/_2$ bunch)

2 tablespoons coarsely chopped fresh basil

$^1/_3$ pound freshly cooked shelled crabmeat or shrimp

2 tablespoons olive oil

1 red onion, finely chopped

1 cup coarsely chopped artichoke hearts

2 cloves garlic, minced

TO PREPARE THE FRITTATA: Whisk the eggs, milk, salt, and pepper together in a large bowl until well blended. Add the bell pepper, spinach, and basil, and stir until incorporated. Gently stir in the crabmeat and set aside.

Heat the olive oil in a 12-inch ovenproof skillet over medium-high heat. Sauté the onion and artichoke hearts until lightly browned, about 5 minutes. Decrease the heat to medium-low and sauté the garlic for about 1 minute. Slowly pour the egg mixture into the skillet and cook until set in the middle but still slightly liquid on the top, 8 to 10 minutes. Meanwhile, preheat the oven broiler and set the rack about 6 inches from the heat source.

Transfer the skillet to the oven and place it under the broiler. Broil the frittata until it is firm on top and golden brown, 5 to 6 minutes. The frittata will rise under the broiler but will deflate quickly when it is removed from the heat. Let the frittata stand at room temperature for 10 minutes before transferring it to a platter and cutting it into wedges.

small bites

These versatile small bites can quell a hungry appetite while dinner is cooking, or provide an elegant starter to a meal. When going out to dinner with friends, we often suggest that everyone gather at our home first for a glass of wine and a few appetizers. Not only does this afford us time to chat, it also brings a personal touch to the evening. The appetizers in this chapter combine well for a cocktail or tapas dinner party and many can be prepared in advance, allowing everyone the opportunity to relax and enjoy the gathering.

spring rolls

Free of `EGG` `NUT` `SUGAR` `OIL*`

MAKES 6 ROLLS

Once you have all the ingredients prepared, assembling these tasty wraps is deliciously fun. The trick to creating beautiful wraps is not using too much filling. Once you've made a couple you will be wrapping like a pro. Spring rolls are incredibly versatile, so after you've mastered these try your own favorite foods for fillings.

12 pieces Pan-Seared Tofu* (page 106), thinly sliced, or packaged gluten-free marinated tofu, if time is short

2 ounces dried bean thread (vermicelli) noodles

1 carrot, peeled and finely julienned

5 green onions, white and green parts, julienned

1 small cucumber, peeled, seeded, and finely julienned

8 fresh mint leaves, slivered (may also use basil or cilantro)

2 tablespoons black sesame seeds, toasted (see page 186)

1 package rice paper wrappers (also called spring roll wrappers)

Tahini Dressing (page 54)

TO PREPARE THE WRAPS: Bring 1 quart of water to a boil in a saucepan. Turn off the heat and add the bean thread noodles. Allow the noodles to soften for about 8 minutes; drain, rinse with cold water, and drain again thoroughly. Cut the noodles into 7-inch lengths and divide into 6 equal portions.

TO MAKE THE ROLLS: Fill a shallow baking pan with warm water. Soak one rice paper wrapper at a time in the warm water until pliable and translucent, 30 seconds to 1 minute. Carefully transfer the rice paper to a clean work surface. Lightly sprinkle with sesame seeds. Layer one-sixth of each of the ingredients on the bottom third of the wrapper. Fold the bottom of the wrapper over the ingredients, fold the sides, and then roll up tightly to enclose the filling. Place the seam-side down on a plate and cover with a damp towel. Continue making the rolls with the remaining ingredients. If making the rolls ahead, place a damp towel over the rolls and wrap the plate in plastic wrap. Keep wrapped and bring to room temperature before serving. Can be made 3 hours ahead.

TO SERVE: Cut the rolls on the diagonal into 1 1/2-inch lengths and arrange on a serving plate. Serve with the Tahini Dressing as a dipping sauce.

shrimp dip *with* belgian endive *and* petite potatoes

Free of | EGG | SOY* | NUT | SUGAR

An attractive presentation and two distinct tastes in one make this appetizer perfect for a party of any size. The creamy shrimp combined with the slightly bitter crisp endive is one way to enjoy this dip, or place a little atop a tender young potato.

8 petite red new potatoes

¹/₃ pound cleaned, cooked shrimp

¹/₃ cup plain dairy-free yogurt* or dairy-free mayonnaise

1¹/₂ teaspoons freshly squeezed lemon juice

¹/₄ cup minced celery (about 1 stalk)

¹/₄ cup red bell pepper, seeded, ribbed, and minced (about ¹/₂ pepper)

2 tablespoons chopped fresh chives (about 1 bunch)

¹/₄ teaspoon salt

¹/₈ teaspoon freshly ground black pepper

4 heads red Belgian endive, leaves separated

4 heads white Belgian endive, leaves separated

TO PREPARE THE POTATOES: In a large pot fitted with a steaming basket, bring water to a boil over medium-high heat. Place the whole potatoes in the steaming basket and cover with a tight-fitting lid. Steam until just tender, 10 to 12 minutes. Do not overcook. Immerse the potatoes in cold water to stop the cooking process and drain. Refrigerate the potatoes until ready to use; they can be made 1 day ahead. Halve the potatoes just before serving.

TO PREPARE THE DIP: Place the shrimp on a plate lined with paper towels. Cover the shrimp with additional paper towels and lightly press out any excess moisture. Combine the yogurt, lemon juice, celery, bell pepper, chives, salt, and pepper in a nonmetallic bowl, and stir to blend. Gently fold in the shrimp until incorporated. Cover with a tight-fitting lid and refrigerate. This dip can be made several hours ahead of serving.

TO ARRANGE THE PLATTER: Transfer the dip to a small bowl with a serving spoon and position the bowl in the corner of a platter. Arrange the potato halves in a half circle around the dip. Next, alternate the red and white endive spears in a half circle around the potatoes, forming a fanned sunburst.

salmon cakes *with* kiwi-papaya salsa

Free of NUT SUGAR

SERVES 6

Serve these irresistible salmon cakes as a starter dish, or to serve them as an appetizer, simply make each cake a bit smaller.

POACHING LIQUID

2 cups water

1 cup dry white wine

1 bay leaf

5 whole black peppercorns

4 sprigs parsley

1/4 cup chopped celery leaves (from about 2 stalks)

SALMON CAKES

1 1/2 pounds salmon steaks or fillets

1/2 cup drained soft tofu (4 ounces)

1 large egg

1/2 cup dairy-free mayonnaise

1/2 teaspoon gluten-free Dijon mustard

1 medium yellow onion, finely chopped

2 tablespoons canola oil, plus more if needed

1 red bell pepper, seeded, ribbed, and finely chopped

1/2 cup finely chopped celery

1/4 cup minced flat-leaf parsley

2 cups Gluten-Free Bread Crumbs (page 185)

Kiwi-Papaya Salsa (page 127)

TO POACH THE SALMON: Combine the water, wine, bay leaf, peppercorns, parsley, and celery leaves in a large sauté pan over medium-high heat. Bring the contents to a boil and add the salmon. Decrease the heat to low, cover, and simmer for 6 to 8 minutes. Transfer the salmon to a plate and set aside to cool. Reserve the poaching liquid.

TO MAKE THE SALMON CAKES: Beat the tofu, egg, mayonnaise, and mustard with an electric mixer in a bowl until creamy, about 2 minutes. Set aside.

In a sauté pan over medium-high heat, sauté the onion in 2 tablespoons of the poaching liquid until softened, about 3 minutes. Transfer the onion to a large bowl and add the bell pepper, celery, and parsley. Flake the salmon into the onion mixture, discarding any bones and skin. Gently fold in the tofu mixture and 1/4 cup of the bread crumbs until just combined.

TO ASSEMBLE AND COOK THE SALMON CAKES: Pour the remaining 1 1/4 cups of bread crumbs on a plate. Using your hands, form the salmon mixture into 18 patties. Place the patties in the bread crumbs and coat them on both sides. Heat the remaining 2 tablespoons of the olive oil over medium heat. Cook the salmon cakes until golden brown, about 2 to 3 minutes per side. Serve immediately topped with the salsa.

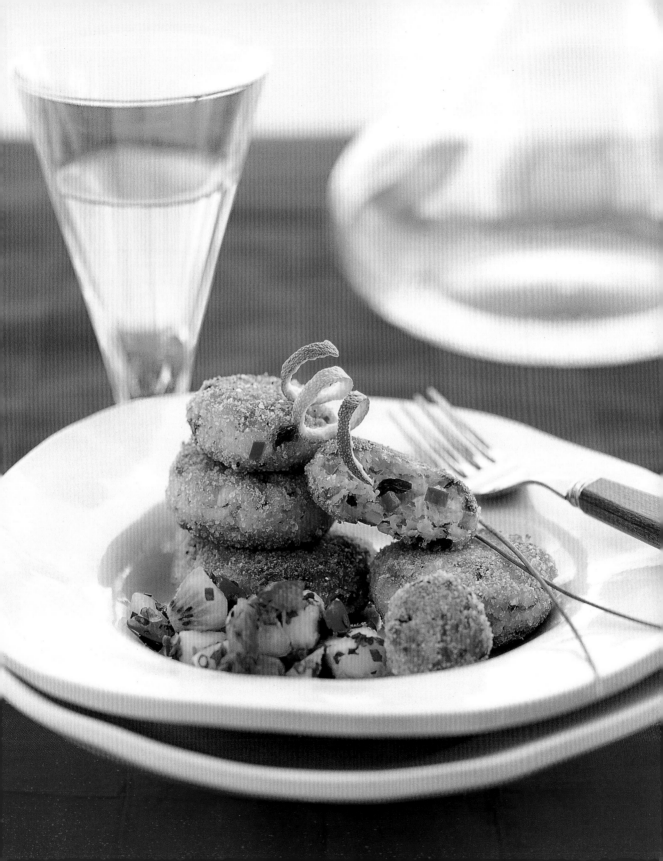

swiss chard *and* almond torta

Free of SOY SUGAR

SERVES 6

These savory bite-size hors d'oeuvres are filled with varied flavors and textures. The combination of chard with fresh herbs adds a healthful flavor to the eggs, while the toasted almonds provide an unexpected finish. Either green or red Swiss chard can be used in this recipe; however, I love the look of the brilliant ruby-red chard alongside the deep green leaves of the basil and parsley.

2 tablespoons olive oil

$^1/_3$ cup Gluten-Free Bread Crumbs (page 185)

2 tablespoons Gluten-Free Flour Mix (page 172)

$^1/_2$ teaspoon gluten-free baking powder

$^1/_2$ teaspoon baking soda

$^1/_4$ teaspoon freshly ground black pepper

$^1/_4$ cup finely chopped almonds, toasted (see page 186)

2 cups finely chopped red onion (about 1 medium onion)

2 cloves garlic, minced

$1^3/_4$ cups finely chopped Swiss chard leaves (4 to 5 stalks)

$^1/_4$ cup chopped fresh basil leaves

2 tablespoons chopped flat-leaf parsley

1 tablespoon chopped fresh dill

4 large eggs

2 teaspoons freshly squeezed lemon juice

Preheat the oven to 300°F. Grease the bottom and sides of an 8 by 8 by 2-inch baking dish with 1 tablespoon of the olive oil. Set aside.

TO PREPARE THE MIXTURE: Combine the bread crumbs, flour, baking powder, baking soda, and pepper in a large bowl. Whisk until blended. Add the almonds and stir to blend.

TO COOK THE TORTA: Heat the remaining tablespoon of olive oil in a large sauté pan over medium-high heat. Add the onion and sauté until it is soft but not brown, about 3 minutes. Add the garlic and Swiss chard, and sauté until the chard is just wilted, 2 to 3 minutes. Remove from the heat and add the basil, parsley, and dill. Add the greens and their liquid to the almond mixture, and toss to coat.

In a small bowl, whisk the eggs and lemon juice together until blended. Stir the egg mixture into the greens until well incorporated. Pour the mixture into the prepared dish and bake until the center is just set, 40 to 45 minutes. Transfer the dish to a wire rack and let cool for about 20 minutes. Slice into 1 to $1^1/_2$-inch bite-size squares.

spanish tortilla

SERVES 4

Vacations are always special, but our trip to Spain was a fun-filled food extravaganza. While staying with our friends Jorge and Blanca, we were treated to one of Blanca's specialties, a marvelous Spanish tortilla. A Spanish tortilla is simply a potato omelet and has nothing in common with its Mexican counterpart. It can be served for brunch, dinner, or as hors d'oeuvres (tapas), hot or at room temperature.

$\frac{1}{4}$ **cup olive oil**

3 pounds russet potatoes, peeled and cut into $\frac{1}{8}$-inch-thick rounds

1 large yellow onion, thinly sliced

5 large eggs

$\frac{1}{4}$ **cup Dairy Milk Alternative (page 173)**

$\frac{1}{4}$ **teaspoon salt**

TO PREPARE THE TORTILLA: Heat 2 tablespoons of the olive oil in an 8- or 9-inch nonstick skillet over medium-low heat. Arrange one-third of the potato slices in a single layer in the skillet. Evenly distribute half of the onions on top of the potato slices, and repeat the layers with one-third potato, the remaining onion, and the remaining potato. Slowly cook the potatoes until they begin to soften, 8 to 10 minutes.

Meanwhile, whisk the eggs, milk, and salt in a bowl until well blended. Decrease the heat to low and pour the egg mixture over the potatoes. Cover and cook the mixture until the egg is slightly firm and the potatoes underneath turn golden brown, about 10 minutes. Uncover, place a large plate upside down on top of the skillet, invert the skillet, and flip the tortilla onto the plate. Return the skillet to medium-low heat, add the remaining 2 tablespoons oil, and slide the tortilla back into the skillet. Cook until golden brown on the other side, about 8 minutes longer. Transfer the tortilla to a platter and allow it to stand at room temperature for 5 minutes before slicing into wedges.

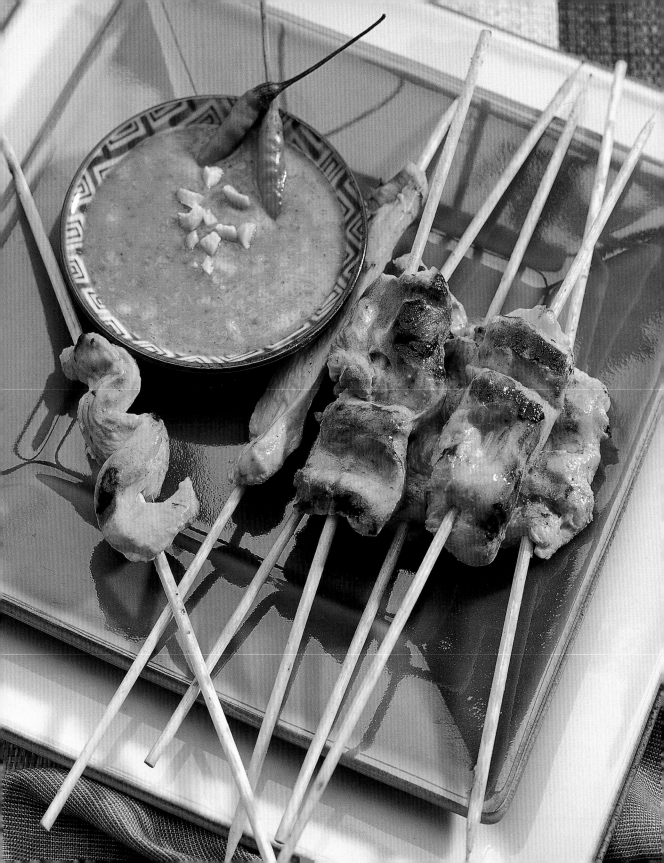

asian chicken skewers
with spicy peanut sauce

SERVES 6

A delectable, easy-to-handle little bite, perfect for entertaining. These Thai-style skewers make a great appetizer. Be sure to have plenty on hand, as they tend to disappear quickly. If you're planning to grill the chicken, wrap the ends of the skewers with a small piece of aluminum foil. In spite of soaking, the skewers will still burn on the grill. Grilling may entail a little more work, but it imparts a wonderful flavor, making it worth the effort.

1 cup unsweetened, canned coconut milk, well blended

$1/3$ cup freshly squeezed lime juice (3 to 4 limes)

3 tablespoons rice vinegar

1 tablespoon ground turmeric

1 tablespoon yellow curry powder

1 tablespoon hot pepper sauce

1 teaspoon salt

4 boneless, skinless chicken breast halves

20 (6-inch) bamboo skewers, soaked in water for 1 hour

Spicy Peanut Sauce (page 123)

TO PREPARE THE MARINADE: Whisk together the coconut milk, lime juice, vinegar, turmeric, curry powder, hot pepper sauce, and salt in a small bowl until well blended. Set aside.

TO MARINATE AND BAKE THE CHICKEN: Cut each chicken breast half lengthwise into about 5 thin strips. Thread each strip of chicken completely onto a skewer, leaving about a $3/4$ inch of the skewer exposed at one end. Place the skewers in a shallow baking dish or in a resealable plastic bag. Pour the marinade over the skewers, covering them completely. Cover and marinate in the refrigerator, turning the skewers occasionally, for about 3 hours or overnight.

Preheat the oven to 425°F. Remove the chicken skewers from the marinade and arrange them on a large, rimmed nonstick baking sheet in a single layer. Discard the marinade. Bake the chicken until just cooked through, about 10 minutes. Transfer the skewers to a platter and serve alongside the peanut sauce.

southwestern fritters

Free of SOY NUT SUGAR

MAKES 2 DOZEN

These colorful little fritters make a terrific party appetizer or a zesty first course served wth a pile of greens tossed in a vinaigrette. The heat from the chiles can vary, so taste before adding them to the mixture, and feel free to add more or less chile according to your liking. If you want to increase the heat, add a little more cayenne pepper to the recipe.

Wear gloves when handling chile peppers, especially jalapeños and habaneros, to prevent your hands from burning and from transferring the capsaicin (the burning compound) to sensitive organs, such as the eyes.

2 large eggs

$1/2$ cup finely chopped red onion (about $1/2$ small onion)

$1/2$ cup finely chopped red bell pepper (about $1/2$ pepper)

$1/2$ cup finely chopped green bell pepper (about $1/2$ pepper)

$1/2$ cup white corn kernels, fresh (about 1 ear) or frozen

2 tablespoons chopped fresh cilantro

2 jalapeño chiles, seeded and minced

2 teaspoons chopped fresh marjoram

$1/2$ teaspoon finely grated lime or lemon zest

$1/2$ teaspoon salt

$1/8$ teaspoon cayenne pepper

7 tablespoons Gluten-Free Bread Crumbs (page 185)

Canola or safflower oil for frying

Pico de Gallo (page 126)

TO MAKE THE BATTER: Whisk the eggs in a large bowl to blend. Add the onion, bell peppers, corn, cilantro, jalapeño, marjoram, zest, salt, cayenne, and bread crumbs and mix until well blended. Set the mixture aside for about 15 minutes to allow the flavors to develop.

TO COOK THE FRITTERS: Line a plate with paper towels. Heat 1 tablespoon oil in a large nonstick skillet over medium-high heat. Using a soupspoon, scoop up approximately 1 tablespoon of the mixture. With the palm of your hand, compact and shape the mixture in the spoon. Gently slide the shaped spoonfuls, about 2 inches in diameter, into the hot oil. Fry until their undersides are golden brown, about 3 minutes. Gently flip the fritters and cook for 3 to 4 minutes longer. Transfer the fritters to the prepared plate to drain. Continue cooking the fritters, adding oil to the pan as needed, 1 tablespoon at a time, with the remaining batter. Serve topped with the Pico de Gallo.

oyster mushrooms rockefeller

Free of SOY SUGAR OIL

SERVES 6

This is a fun spin on an old-time classic. I served this at a dinner party and it was a huge success. The various textures—soft, creamy, and crunchy— offer a little something for everyone.

$^1/_2$ cup cashew pieces

2 cups finely chopped fresh spinach, tightly packed (about 1 bunch)

$^3/_4$ pound fresh oyster mushrooms, tough parts of the stem removed

$^1/_2$ cup Gluten-Free Bread Crumbs (page 185)

$^1/_3$ cup minced fennel bulb or celery (about $^1/_2$ bulb)

$^1/_4$ cup minced yellow onion (about $^1/_2$ small onion)

2 cloves garlic, minced

2 tablespoons chopped flat-leaf parsley

$^1/_4$ teaspoon salt

$^1/_3$ cup water

$^1/_4$ cup freshly squeezed lemon juice (about 1 lemon)

2 teaspoons Dijon mustard

$^1/_8$ teaspoon hot pepper sauce, or to taste

In a small bowl soak the cashews in enough cold water to cover. Set aside.

Meanwhile, set 6 ovenproof, $^1/_2$-cup ramekins on a baking sheet and distribute the mushrooms equally in the bottom of each ramekin. In a large sauté pan over medium-high heat, add $^1/_4$ cup of water and the spinach and sauté until the spinach is wilted and the water has just evaporated, about 3 minutes. Distribute the wilted spinach equally on top of the mushrooms.

TO PREPARE THE TOPPING AND BAKE THE DISH: Preheat the oven to 400°F. In a bowl combine the bread crumbs, fennel, onion, garlic, parsley, and salt; stir to blend. Drain the cashews in a fine-mesh strainer and rinse under cold running water; drain again. Place the cashews, water, lemon juice, mustard, and hot pepper sauce in a blender. Cover the blender and whirl at top speed until the mixture is smooth and creamy, scraping down the sides as need, about 2 minutes. Add half of the cashew mixture to the bread mixture, tossing until incorporated and the mixture is uniformly moist. Evenly distribute the mixture on top of the spinach and top each ramekin with 1 tablespoon of the cashew mixture. Bake for 15 minutes. Set the oven to broil, move the ramekins under the broiler, and cook until the cashew cream is lightly brown, 2 to 3 minutes. Serve warm.

scallop-prosciutto bundles

Free of EGG SOY NUT SUGAR OIL*

SERVES 4

There's so much visual drama in these elegant little bundles that they can be served as a fabulous first course or even as a light meal. The width of the prosciutto will determine how many slices you'll need.

$^1/_3$ cup dry white wine

$^1/_4$ cup freshly squeezed lemon juice (about 2 lemons)

2 green onions, white and green parts, minced

8 whole black peppercorns

1 bay leaf

12 fresh jumbo scallops

1 bunch fresh chives

6 to 12 paper-thin slices prosciutto

Freshly squeezed lemon juice

$1^1/_2$ cups finely shredded green cabbage (about $^1/_2$ small head)

Olive oil* (optional)

Balsamic vinegar

Freshly ground black pepper

Lemon wedges, for garnish (optional)

TO POACH THE SCALLOPS: Combine the wine, lemon juice, green onion, peppercorns, and bay leaf in a large sauté pan over medium-high heat. Bring to a boil, add the scallops, and decrease the heat to medium-low. Cook the scallops for 2 to 3 minutes, turning once, until just heated through.

TO PREPARE THE CHIVES: Fill a bowl with ice water and set aside. Bring a pot of water to a boil and immerse the chives for 6 seconds. Quickly transfer the chives to the ice bath for 15 seconds, then transfer to a paper towel to drain.

TO ASSEMBLE: Place 1 slice of prosciutto on a flat work surface. Place a scallop at one end and gently roll up in the prosciutto. Place the wrapped scallop in the center of a chive and tie around the bundle, as if wrapping a package. Continue until all the scallops are wrapped.

Place a large nonstick skillet over medium-high heat. Transfer the bundles to the hot skillet and sprinkle with lemon juice. Cover, and cook until the prosciutto begins to look transparent, about 4 minutes.

Divide the cabbage equally among 4 individual plates and sprinkle with olive oil, vinegar, and pepper. Arrange 3 bundles on each plate, and garnish with a lemon wedge. Serve warm.

salads and dressings

The dressings in this chapter embody a light, creamy, smooth texture and can be prepared in no time. When making dressing that contains oil, a good rule of thumb is to mix 3 parts oil to 1 part vinegar. If you have the time, make a dressing 2 to 24 hours in advance to allow the flavors time to fully blend. Also, be sure to mix the dressing well and taste and correct the seasonings *before* you toss it with a salad.

mixed greens *with* citrus *and* candied pecans

Free of EGG*

SERVES 6

I prepared this salad for 120 ladies at a spring luncheon and it got rave reviews. It's light, colorful, and refreshing, with the tangy grapefruit providing a nice contrast to the sweet candied pecans. Markets now carry an assortment of mixed greens in bulk or prewashed in bags, making it convenient to add variety to your salads.

DRESSING

$1/3$ cup dairy-free mayonnaise

2 tablespoons freshly squeezed lemon juice

$1/4$ cup freshly squeezed orange juice

1 tablespoon rice vinegar

$1/2$ teaspoon balsamic vinegar

1 tablespoon Orange Date Syrup (page 189) or honey

2 tablespoons freshly squeezed lemon juice

$1/4$ teaspoon salt

$1/4$ teaspoon freshly ground black pepper

SALAD

2 ruby grapefruits

2 heads romaine hearts, torn into bite-size pieces

4 cups mixed greens (an assortment of frisée, radicchio, arugula, escarole, and watercress)

$3/4$ cup Candied Pecans* (page 188)

TO PREPARE THE DRESSING: Whisk together the mayonnaise, lemon juice, orange juice, vinegars, date syrup, salt, and pepper in a small bowl until well blended. Taste and correct the seasonings. Cover and refrigerate for 1 hour or up to 5 days.

TO PREPARE THE GRAPEFRUIT: Peel the grapefruits and remove all of the white pith. Working over a bowl, cut the grapefruit between the membranes to release the segments. Spoon 2 tablespoons of the dressing over the grapefruit segments to coat. Let stand for 15 minutes or up to 1 hour.

TO ASSEMBLE THE SALAD: Toss the greens in a large bowl until well combined. Pour the remaining dressing over the greens, and toss to coat. Divide the greens equally among 6 plates. Arrange the grapefruit segments on top of the greens, and scatter the pecans on top. Serve immediately.

the dairy-free and gluten-free kitchen

panzanella salad

Free of SOY NUT SUGAR

SERVES 4 TO 6

This Tuscan bread salad is one of my all-time favorites when summer tomatoes are at their peak. Pick any of the beefsteak heirloom varieties, such as Brandywine, Marvel Striped, Cherokee Purple, Evergreen, or Goldie; any combination would be amazing in this salad.

1 medium red onion, thinly sliced

2 tablespoons extra virgin olive oil

1/4 cup balsamic vinegar

1 clove garlic, minced

1/2 teaspoon kosher salt

1/4 teaspoon freshly ground black pepper

3 pounds beefsteak tomatoes

1 tablespoon drained capers

6 slices Fiber-Rich Sandwich Bread, cut 1 inch thick (page 137)

1 English cucumber, peeled, seeded, and sliced

1/2 cup packed fresh basil leaves, chopped

TO PREPARE THE SALAD: Immerse the sliced onion in a bowl of cold water and swish it occasionally to release some of its sharp, acidic flavor, about 10 minutes. Drain the water and refill the bowl with fresh water. Repeat the process until the onion has soaked for about 30 minutes. Drain the onion and blot it dry with paper towels. Meanwhile, combine the olive oil, vinegar, garlic, salt, and pepper in a large nonmetallic bowl and whisk to blend. Add the onions, tomatoes, capers, and toss to combine. Set aside.

TO PREPARE THE BREAD AND ASSEMBLE THE SALAD: Place the bread on a hot 350°F grill or on a sheet pan under a heated broiler and toast both sides until dry but not hard, 2 to 3 minutes. Tear the bread by hand into 1-inch pieces and add it to the tomato mixture. Add the cucumber and basil, and toss to incorporate. Serve family style.

sweet *and* tangy jicama slaw

Free of EGG SOY* NUT SUGAR OIL*

SERVES 4 TO 6

Crunchy jicama is a nice addition to this summer-time classic, adding a unique texture and flavor not found in common coleslaw. Jicama's cool crispness pairs beautifully with grilled meats, or use it as a topping for Shrimp Tacos (page 73).

DRESSING

¹/₃ cup dairy-free mayonnaise or plain dairy-free yogurt*

2 tablespoons freshly squeezed lime juice

2 tablespoons rice vinegar

2 tablespoons Date Syrup (page 189) or honey

¹/₄ teaspoon salt

¹/₈ teaspoon freshly ground black pepper

SALAD

4 cups shredded green cabbage (1 one-pound head)

2 cups peeled, sliced jicama, in 1¹/₂-inch julienne (about 1 small jicama)

2 carrots, peeled and cut into 1¹/₂-inch julienne

1 red bell pepper, seeded, ribbed, and cut into 1¹/₂-inch julienne

¹/₂ cup coarsely chopped green onion, white and green parts (about ¹/₂ bunch)

¹/₃ cup chopped flat-leaf parsley (about ¹/₂ bunch)

TO PREPARE THE DRESSING: Whisk together the mayonnaise, lime juice, vinegar, sugar, salt, and pepper in a small bowl until well blended. Set aside.

TO ASSEMBLE THE SALAD: Combine the cabbage, jicama, carrot, green onion, and parsley in a large bowl. Toss to mix. Pour the dressing over the salad and toss until well incorporated. Taste and correct the seasonings. Cover and refrigerate for 1 to 3 hours. Toss the salad again before serving.

red sea potato salad

SERVES 6

This Middle Eastern-style dressing goes a long way in flavoring this potato salad while giving it a high-protein boost to boot! Serve it alongside vegetables for a delightful summer meal or pair it with grilled favorites off the barbeque. If red new potatoes are not available, choose any low-starch white fleshed potato such as Katahdin, Superior, Chippewa, White Rose, La Rouge, Red La Soda, or Red Pontiac.

DRESSING

- ³/₄ cup plain dairy-free yogurt*
- ¹/₂ cup Zesty Lemon Hummus (page 128)
- 3 tablespoons Dairy Milk Alternative (page 173)

SALAD

- 2 pounds red new potatoes
- 1 cup chopped celery
- ¹/₂ cup red onion, finely chopped
- ¹/₄ cup chopped flat-leaf parsley
- 2 tablespoon capers, drained, and rinsed

TO PREPARE THE DRESSING: Stir together the yogurt, hummus, and milk in a small bowl until blended. Set aside.

TO PREPARE THE ONION: Immerse the chopped onion in a bowl of cold water and swish it occasionally to release some of its sharp, acidic flavor, about 10 minutes. Drain the onion and blot it dry with paper towels.

TO PREPARE THE POTATOES: Place the potatoes in a large pot with enough water to cover them by 2 inches. Bring the water to a boil and cook the potatoes until just tender, about 20 minutes. Drain the potatoes in a colander and rinse under cold water until the potatoes are cool enough to handle.

TO ASSEMBLE THE SALAD: Cut the potatoes into 1-inch pieces and place them in a large bowl. Add the celery, onion, parsley, and capers. Add the dressing to the potatoes and gently toss until just incorporated. Serve at room temperature.

spinach, pear, *and* beet salad *with* sherry dressing

Free of | EGG | SOY | NUT | SUGAR

SERVES 4 TO 6

This winter salad makes an ideal starter for a holiday dinner. The tender, dark green spinach, earthy beets, slightly sweet pear, and crimson cranberries give this salad a complexity of textures, colors, and flavors. For salads, I prefer the flavor of baked beets to boiled. The baking process makes them incredibly sweet while retaining their natural flavor.

SALAD

3 medium golden or red beets, trimmed

6 cups stemmed baby spinach leaves, lightly packed (about 1 bunch)

3 ripe Bartlett or Bosc pears, peeled, cored, and cut into 1/4-inch-thick slices

1/3 cup dried cranberries

DRESSING

1 cup peeled, cored, and diced ripe Bartlett or Bosc pear (1 or 2 pears)

1/3 cup dry sherry

1/4 cup olive oil

2 tablespoons freshly squeezed lemon juice

1 small shallot, chopped

1 teaspoon gluten-free Dijon mustard

1 teaspoon Date Syrup (page 189) or honey

1/4 teaspoon salt

1/8 teaspoon freshly ground black pepper

TO PREPARE THE BEETS: Preheat the oven to 425°F. Wrap the beets individually in aluminum foil, enclosing them completely. Roast the beets in the oven for about 1 hour and 15 minutes, or until tender when pierced with a fork. Allow the beets to cool completely, about 2 hours or overnight. Using a sharp paring knife, peel the beets and slice them 1/2 inch thick. Meanwhile, prepare the dressing.

TO PREPARE THE DRESSING: Combine the diced pear, sherry, olive oil, lemon juice, shallot, mustard, date syrup, salt, and pepper in a blender and puree until smooth. Taste and correct the seasonings.

TO ASSEMBLE THE SALAD: Place the spinach in a large bowl. Pour the dressing over the greens and toss to coat. Divide the greens equally among 4 to 6 plates. Arrange the pear slices and beets atop the greens, and scatter the cranberries over them. Serve immediately.

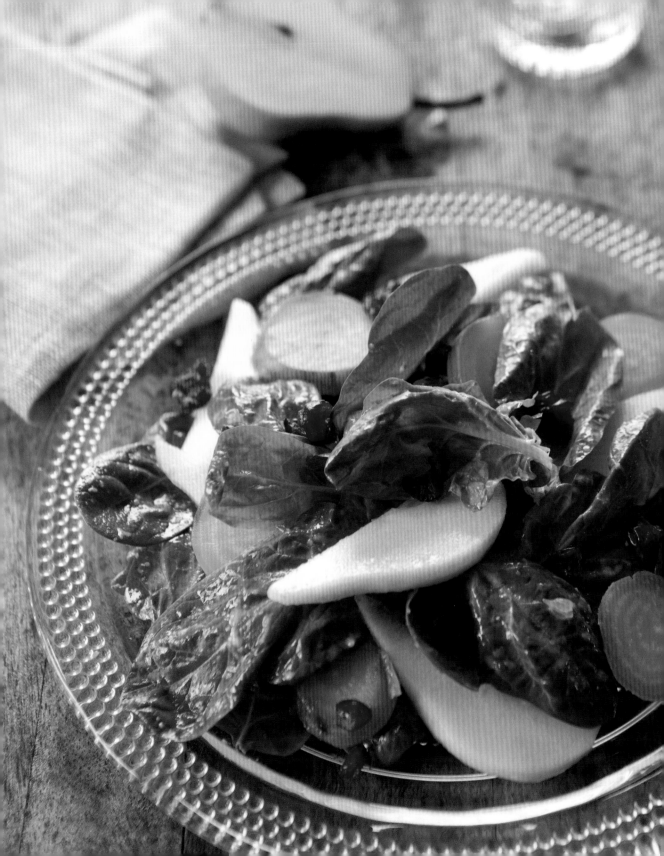

chicken salad

Free of EGG · SOY* · SUGAR · OIL

SERVES 6

This salad is as delicious as it is pretty and makes a terrific luncheon main course. I like to serve it tumbling out of a split Orange Popover (page 139) resting on a bed of butter lettuce. Steeping the chicken breasts produces tender and succulent meat that is ideal for a salad. As an alternative, roast chicken with the skin and bones removed also works well. Figure on one 2-pound roast chicken yielding about 4 cups of cubed or shredded meat.

SALAD

4 boneless, skinless chicken breast halves, about 6 ounces each

1 cup thinly sliced celery (about 3 stalks)

1/2 cup thinly sliced green onion, white and green parts (about 1/2 bunch)

1 cup red seedless grapes

1/2 cup pecan halves, toasted (see page 186)

2 tablespoons chopped flat-leaf parsley

DRESSING

3/4 cup plain dairy-free yogurt*

3 tablespoons apple cider vinegar

1 tablespoon Date Syrup (page 189) or honey

1 tablespoon poppyseeds

1/2 teaspoon salt

1/4 teaspoon ground white pepper

TO PREPARE THE CHICKEN: Fill a stockpot with water and bring to a boil over high heat. Add the chicken to the boiling water, cover, and return to a boil. Boil the chicken for 2 to 3 minutes. Turn off the heat, and let the chicken steep, covered, until it is no longer pink in the thickest part of the breast, 10 to 15 minutes. Using a slotted spoon, transfer the chicken to a plate and let cool for approximately 20 minutes. Meanwhile, prepare the dressing.

TO PREPARE THE DRESSING AND ASSEMBLE THE SALAD: Whisk together the yogurt, vinegar, date syrup, poppyseeds, salt, and pepper in a large bowl until well blended. Cut the cooked, cooled breast meat into 3/4-inch cubes; you should have about 4 cups. Add the chicken, celery, green onion, grapes, pecans, and parsley to the dressing. Toss to coat. Taste and correct the seasonings. Serve immediately.

asian peanut pasta salad

SERVES 6

This Asian-influenced chilled noodle salad is a success at parties, pleasing adults and kids alike. It can be served as a starter but makes a fantastic main course as well. The addition of Pan-Seared Tofu (page 106) adds a substantial amount of protein as well as delicious flavor from its marinade.

1 (12-ounce) package gluten-free spaghetti

1 tablespoon dark sesame oil

4 cups shredded napa cabbage (about one 1-pound head)

1 red bell pepper, seeded, ribbed, and cut into $1^1/_2$-inch julienne

2 carrots, peeled and cut into $1^1/_2$-inch julienne

2 tablespoons chopped flat-leaf parsley

4 green onions, white and green parts, thinly sliced

1 cup Spicy Peanut Sauce (page 123)

Pan-Seared Tofu (page 106), chilled and cut into $^1/_2$-inch cubes, or packaged gluten-free marinated tofu

TO COOK THE SPAGHETTI: Bring 3 quarts of water to a boil in a large saucepan over high heat. Add the pasta to the water. Allow the water to return to a boil and stir. Cook the pasta, uncovered, according to the package directions, taking care not to overcook it. Drain the pasta in a colander, rinse under cold running water, and drain again. Transfer the pasta to a large bowl and toss with the sesame oil to coat.

TO ASSEMBLE THE SALAD: Place the cabbage, bell pepper, carrot, parsley, and green onion in a large bowl. Pour the peanut sauce over the vegetables and toss to coat. Add the pasta and tofu and gently toss until well combined. Serve immediately, or cover and refrigerate for up to 1 day. If refrigerated, bring to room temperature before serving.

black bean *and* corn salad

Free of EGG SOY NUT SUGAR

SERVES 6

This colorful salad is perfect for summer gatherings. It is quick and easy to prepare, keeps well, and tastes great too. The combination of tender black beans, crunchy red peppers, rich avocado, refreshing cilantro, and sweet corn is a delight to the palate. I prefer using fresh white corn to yellow because I find it to be sweeter and more tender; however, yellow corn works equally well.

DRESSING

2 tablespoons rice wine vinegar

1 tablespoon Date Syrup (page 189) or honey

1 tablespoon olive oil

$^1/_2$ teaspoon freshly squeezed lemon juice

$^1/_4$ teaspoon salt

$^1/_8$ teaspoon freshly ground black pepper

SALAD

$^1/_2$ cup finely chopped red onion (about $^1/_2$ small onion)

2 cups white corn kernels, fresh (4 to 6 ears) or frozen

4 cups cooked (see page 180) or canned black beans, rinsed well

1 red bell pepper, seeded, ribbed, and chopped into $^1/_4$-inch pieces

$^1/_3$ cup minced fresh cilantro

1 ripe avocado, diced

TO PREPARE THE DRESSING: Whisk together the vinegar, date syrup, olive oil, lemon juice, salt, and pepper in a small bowl until blended. Set aside.

TO PREPARE THE ONION: Immerse the chopped onion in a bowl of cold water and swish it occasionally to release some of its sharp, acidic flavor, about 10 minutes. Drain the water and refill the bowl with fresh water. Repeat the process until the onion has soaked for about 30 minutes. Drain the onion and blot it dry with paper towels.

TO ASSEMBLE THE SALAD: Place the beans, corn, onion, and bell pepper in a large bowl and toss to mix. Add the dressing to the bean mixture and gently toss until just incorporated. Cover and refrigerate for about 2 hours. Add the avocado and cilantro and gently toss again before serving.

rainbow quinoa salad

Free of EGG SOY NUT SUGAR OIL

SERVES 6

A mandoline makes creating this beautiful salad a breeze. The combination of raw vegetables with the colorful quinoa (pronounced keen-WAH) is a feast for the eyes. If you cannot find black or red quinoa the yellow will work just fine. Although it is a seed, quinoa is referred to as a "super grain" because it contains all eight essential amino acids, making it a good protein source. Soaking and washing the quinoa is an important step; it removes and rinses away a bitter coating, thus sweetening the grain.

SALAD

3/4 **cup yellow quinoa**

1/4 **cup black or red quinoa**

2 **cups water**

2 **zucchini, julienned**

2 **yellow squash, julienned**

2 **carrots, julienned**

1 **cup cherry tomatoes, halved**

2 **green onions chopped, white and green parts**

1/4 **cup minced flat-leaf parsley**

1/2 **cup Sweet Vinaigrette (page 52)**

TO PREPARE THE QUINOA: Place the quinoa in a bowl and cover with cold water, soak for 15 minutes. Place your hand in the bowl and massage the quinoa thoroughly; the water will become cloudy. Pour the quinoa into a fine-mesh strainer; drain, rinse under cold running water, and drain again. In a saucepan over medium-high heat bring the water to a boil. Add the quinoa, decrease the heat to low, cover, and simmer for 20 minutes. Set aside to cool. Once cool, fluff with a fork.

TO ASSEMBLE THE SALAD: In a large bowl add the quinoa, zucchini, yellow squash, and carrots, tossing to combine. Add the tomatoes, onion, parsley, and vinaigrette. Gently toss to combine and serve.

sweet vinaigrette

MAKES ¹/₂ CUP

3 tablespoons Date Syrup or Orange Date Syrup (page 189)

2 tablespoons apple cider vinegar

¹/₄ teaspoon salt

¹/₈ teaspoon freshly ground black pepper

TO PREPARE THE VINAIGRETTE: In a small bowl combine the date syrup, vinegar, salt, and pepper, whisking to blend. Set aside. Transfer the dressing to a container with a tight-fitting lid, cover, and refrigerate for at least 2 hours or overnight. Before serving, mix to blend, and taste and correct the seasonings. The dressing will keep for 5 days in the refrigerator, tightly covered.

creamy papaya vinaigrette

MAKES 1¹/₂ CUPS

1 ripe papaya, peeled, seeded, and cut into quarters

¹/₄ cup vanilla Dairy Milk Alternative (page 173)

3 tablespoons freshly squeezed lime juice (about 2 limes)

2 tablespoons dairy-free mayonnaise* or plain soy yogurt

2 tablespoons apple cider vinegar

¹/₄ teaspoon salt

TO PREPARE THE DRESSING: Place the papaya, milk, lime juice, mayonnaise, vinegar, and salt in a blender. Whirl at top speed until smooth, about 1 minute. Transfer the dressing to a container with a tight-fitting lid; cover and refrigerate for at least 2 hours or overnight. Before serving, whisk the dressing to blend, and taste and correct the seasonings. The dressing will keep for 5 days in the refrigerator, tightly covered.

summer fruit salad dressing

Free of EGG SOY NUT SUGAR OIL

MAKES 1¹/₂ CUPS

¹/₄ cup freshly squeezed lime juice (2 to 3 limes)

1 teaspoon minced lime zest

1 tablespoon minced fresh cilantro

3 tablespoons freshly squeezed orange juice

TO PREPARE THE DRESSING: Whisk together the lime juice, zest, cilantro, and orange juice in a small bowl until blended. This dressing is best served immediately.

creamy avocado dressing

Free of EGG NUT SUGAR OIL

MAKES 1¹/₄ CUPS

1 ripe avocado, halved

¹/₂ cup Dairy Milk Alternative (page 173)

2 tablespoons freshly squeezed lemon juice

2 green onions, white and green parts, chopped

1 tablespoon white or yellow miso

¹/₂ teaspoon fresh dill, or ¹/₄ teaspoon dried

¹/₈ teaspoon ground white pepper

TO PREPARE THE DRESSING: Combine the avocado, milk, lemon juice, onion, miso, dill, and pepper in a blender. Whirl at top speed until smooth, about 1 minute, scraping down the sides with a rubber spatula. Transfer the dressing to a container with a tight-fitting lid; cover and refrigerate for at least 2 hours or overnight. Before serving, mix to blend, and taste and correct the seasonings. Thin with additional milk if desired. This dressing will keep for 5 days in the refrigerator, tightly covered.

creamy tarragon dressing

Free of EGG SOY* NUT SUGAR

MAKES 1 CUP

¹/₄ cup white wine vinegar

¹/₃ cup extra virgin olive oil

3 tablespoons minced fresh tarragon

2 tablespoons minced fresh chives

1 clove garlic, minced

1 tablespoon gluten-free Dijon mustard

2 tablespoons dairy-free mayonnaise*

1 teaspoon Date Syrup (page 189) or honey

¹/₈ teaspoon salt

¹/₈ teaspoon freshly ground black pepper

Whisk together all the ingredients in a bowl. Transfer the dressing to a container with a tight-fitting lid, cover, and refrigerate for at least 2 hours or overnight. Before serving, mix to blend, and taste and correct the seasonings. The dressing will keep for 5 days in the refrigerator, tightly covered.

tahini dressing

Free of EGG NUT SUGAR OIL

MAKES ¹/₂ CUP

2 tablespoons tahini

¹/₄ cup rice vinegar

2 teaspoons gluten-free tamari

4 cloves garlic, minced

1 tablespoon Date Syrup (page 189) or maple syrup

1 tablespoon freshly squeezed lime or lemon juice

1 Thai chile pepper or jalapeño, finely chopped (optional)

Combine the tahini, vinegar, tamari, garlic, date syrup, lime juice, and chile in a bowl. Whisk together until well blended. Transfer the dressing to a container with a tight-fitting lid; cover and refrigerate for at least 2 hours or overnight. Before serving, whisk the dressing to blend. The dressing will keep for 5 days in the refrigerator, tightly covered.

soups

Once you have a few fundamental techniques established, whipping up a nurturing bowl of soup becomes effortless. You can double a recipe and freeze the extra in small batches. I line a measuring cup with a heavy, self-sealing plastic freezer bag, making it easy to store the exact amount for a meal. Many of the soups in this chapter are so luscious and creamy, if you hadn't made them yourself, you would think they were made with heavy cream. Any of the vegetable soups that use chicken stock as the base can become vegan simply by preparing them with vegetable stock.

carrot *and* roasted red pepper soup

SERVES 6

Rich and vibrant in color with a lightly roasted flavor, this soup makes a wonderful first course. It can be prepared up to 2 days in advance. Allow the soup to cool, then refrigerate it in a tightly sealed container. Rewarm the soup over low heat, stirring occasionally, until hot.

1 pound carrots, peeled and cut into 2-inch pieces

2 large red bell peppers, roasted (see page 182) and cut into quarters

1 large yellow onion, coarsely chopped

2$^{1}/_{2}$ cups Chicken Stock (page 176) or Vegetable Stock (page 177)

$^{3}/_{4}$ cup dry white wine

$^{1}/_{8}$ teaspoon ground cumin

$^{1}/_{2}$ teaspoon salt

$^{1}/_{8}$ teaspoon freshly ground black pepper

$^{3}/_{4}$ cup Dairy Milk Alternative (page 173), plus more if needed

1 tablespoon minced roasted red bell pepper, for garnish (optional)

TO PREPARE THE SOUP: In a saucepan, combine the carrots, roasted peppers, onion, stock, white wine, cumin, salt, and pepper. Bring to a boil. Cover, decrease the heat, and simmer until the vegetables are tender when pierced with a fork, about 25 minutes.

TO PUREE THE SOUP: Remove the soup from the heat and ladle half of it into a blender, along with $^{1}/_{2}$ cup of the milk. Puree until smooth. Empty the blender into a large bowl and repeat with the remaining soup and $^{1}/_{4}$ cup of milk. Transfer the pureed soup back to the saucepan. Thin the soup if necessary by adding a little more milk, $^{1}/_{4}$ cup at a time, until the desired consistency is achieved. Taste and correct the seasonings. Reheat over low heat, stirring occasionally, until heated through, taking care not to boil the soup. Ladle into bowls, and garnish with a sprinkling of minced roasted pepper.

yukon gold potato-leek soup

Free of EGG SOY NUT SUGAR OIL

SERVES 6

Incredibly rich in flavor and luxurious to the palate, Yukon Gold potatoes lend themselves nicely to this comforting classic. Leeks may look like overgrown green onions but their flavor is milder and sweeter than other alliums, such as onions and garlic.

4 medium leeks, white and pale green parts only, sliced 1 inch thick

2$^{1}/_{2}$ cups Chicken Stock (page 176) or Vegetable Stock (page 177)

1$^{1}/_{2}$ pounds Yukon Gold potatoes, peeled and cut into 2-inch pieces

$^{1}/_{2}$ teaspoon salt

$^{1}/_{8}$ teaspoon ground white pepper

1$^{1}/_{4}$ cups Dairy Milk Alternative (page 173), plus more if needed

$^{1}/_{2}$ bunch chives cut into 2-inch-long pieces, for garnish (optional)

TO PREPARE THE SOUP: Heat a large saucepan over medium-high heat and add the leeks and 2 tablespoons of stock; steam-saute, stirring frequently, until the leeks are soft but not brown, about 3 minutes. Add the chicken stock, potatoes, salt, and pepper; bring to a boil. Cover, decrease the heat to low, and simmer until the vegetables are tender when pierced with a fork, about 20 minutes.

TO PUREE THE SOUP: Remove the soup from the heat and ladle half of it into a blender, along with $^{3}/_{4}$ cup of the milk. Cover and puree until smooth. Empty the blender into a large bowl and repeat with the remaining soup and $^{1}/_{2}$ cup of milk. Transfer the pureed soup back to the saucepan. Thin the soup if necessary by adding a little more milk, $^{1}/_{4}$ cup at a time, until the desired consistency is achieved. Taste and correct the seasonings. Reheat over low heat, stirring occasionally, until heated through, taking care not to boil the soup. Ladle the soup into bowls and garnish with the chives.

butternut squash *and* pear soup

Free of EGG SOY NUT SUGAR OIL

SERVES 6

This soup, bright tasting with a lovely color, is delicious served during the fall and winter months. The fresh pears provide a slightly sweet background flavor. For a simple yet satisfying meal, serve it alongside a salad of tart greens and Rosemary Drop Biscuits (page 144).

2$^{1}/_{2}$ **pounds butternut squash, peeled, seeded, and cut into** $^{1}/_{2}$**-inch pieces (about 6 cups)**

1 medium onion, coarsely chopped

3$^{1}/_{2}$ **cups Chicken Stock (page 176) or Vegetable Stock (page 177)**

2 Bosc pears, peeled, cored, and cut into 2-inch pieces

1 teaspoon freshly squeezed lemon juice

$^{1}/_{2}$ **teaspoon salt**

1 cup Dairy Milk Alternative (page 173), plus more if needed

Minced fresh parsley, for garnish (optional)

TO PREPARE THE SOUP: Heat a large saucepan over medium-high heat. Add the butternut squash, onion, and 2 tablespoons of stock, and steam-sauté, stirring frequently, until softened but not brown about 10 minutes. If the vegetables begin to stick to the pan, add 2 tablespoons more stock. Add the remaining stock, pears, lemon juice, and salt. Bring to a boil. Cover and decrease the heat to low. Simmer until the vegetables are tender when pierced with a fork, about 25 minutes.

TO PUREE THE SOUP: Remove the soup from the heat and ladle half of it into a blender along with $^{1}/_{2}$ cup of the milk. Cover and puree until smooth. Empty the blender and repeat with the remaining soup and the remaining $^{1}/_{2}$ cup of milk. Transfer the pureed soup back to the saucepan. Thin the soup if necessary by adding a little more milk, $^{1}/_{4}$ cup at a time, until the desired consistency is achieved. Taste and correct the seasonings. Reheat over low heat, stirring occasionally, until hot, taking care not to boil the soup. Ladle into bowls and garnish with minced parsley.

white bean vegetable soup

Free of EGG SOY NUT SUGAR OIL

SERVES 6

This Tuscan-style soup, with its healthful combination of calcium-rich vegetables and beans, takes the chill off cold winter days. I prefer using small white navy beans, but cannellini and lima beans are also delicious. Enjoy it with a warm slice of Sweet Potato Cornbread (page 145) or Amaranth Sesame Breadsticks (page 143).

1 large yellow onion, coarsely chopped

3 cloves garlic, minced

$^1/_2$ small butternut squash, peeled, seeded, and cut into $^1/_2$-inch pieces

3 carrots, peeled, sliced lengthwise, and cut into $^1/_2$-inch pieces

2 stalks celery, cut into $^1/_4$-inch dice

5 cups Chicken Stock (page 176) or Vegetable Stock (page 177)

$1^1/_4$-cups Chopped Tomatoes (page 179)

2 large sage leaves, chopped, or $^1/_4$ tablespoon minced fresh parsley

$^1/_2$ teaspoon dried sage, crumbled

1 teaspoon salt

$^1/_8$ teaspoon freshly ground black pepper

1 bunch kale, stemmed and finely chopped

2 cups cooked white beans (see page 188)

TO PREPARE THE SOUP: Heat a large saucepan over medium-high heat and add the onion and 2 tablespoons of the stock, stirring frequently, until the onion is tender, about 3 minutes. Add the garlic and cook another 30 seconds without letting it brown. Add the squash, carrot, celery, stock, tomato, sage, parsley, salt, and pepper. Bring to a boil. Cover and decrease the heat to low. Simmer the vegetables until tender, about 20 minutes. Add the kale and beans and continue cooking for 10 minutes longer, stirring occasionally, to allow the flavors to fully develop. Ladle the soup into bowls and serve.

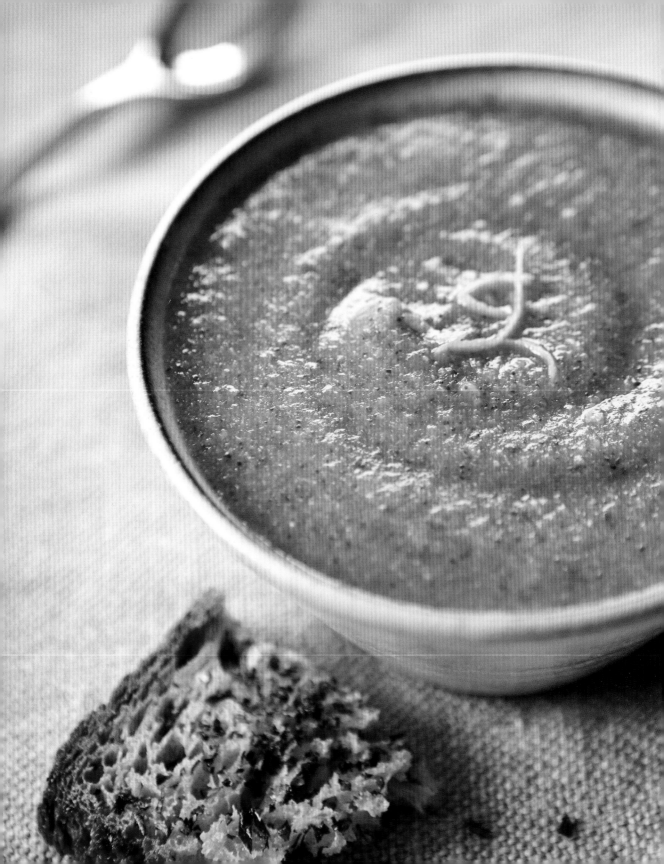

creamy broccoli soup

Free of EGG SOY NUT SUGAR OIL

SERVES 6

This mild, creamy soup is enhanced with just a hint of lemon. It's the only way I can get my husband to eat and enjoy broccoli. Not only does this soup taste great, but broccoli is a calcium-rich vegetable, and this soup is loaded with it.

2 pounds broccoli, stems and florets chopped separately into 1-inch pieces

1 large yellow onion, coarsely chopped

1¹/₂ pounds russet potatoes, peeled and cut into 2-inch pieces (about 2 potatoes)

3¹/₂ cups Chicken Stock (page 176) or Vegetable Stock (page 177)

¹/₄ teaspoon freshly squeezed lemon juice

2 bay leaves

¹/₂ teaspoon salt

¹/₈ teaspoon freshly ground black pepper

³/₄ cup Dairy Milk Alternative (page 173), plus more if needed

Herb Toast (page 185), for garnish (optional)

Grated lemon zest, for garnish (optional)

TO PREPARE THE SOUP: Combine the broccoli stems, onion, potatoes, stock, lemon juice, bay leaves, salt, and pepper in a large saucepan. Bring to a boil. Cover, decrease the heat to low, and simmer until the vegetables are tender, about 15 minutes. Raise the heat to medium-high and bring to a boil. Add broccoli florets; reduce the heat to low, and simmer until florets are just tender, about 8 minutes. (By placing the broccoli florets on top of the other partially cooked vegetables, they cook via steam, and retain their vibrant green color.)

TO PUREE THE SOUP: Remove the soup from the heat and discard the bay leaves. Ladle half of the soup into a blender along with ¹/₂ cup of the milk, cover, and puree until smooth. Empty the blender into a large bowl and repeat with the remaining soup and ¹/₄ cup of milk. Transfer the pureed soup back to the saucepan. Thin the soup if necessary by adding a little more milk, ¹/₄ cup at a time, until the desired consistency is achieved. Taste and correct the seasonings. Reheat over low heat, stirring occasionally, until heated through, taking care not to boil the soup. Ladle into bowls and garnish with Herb Toast (page 185) and lemon zest.

three mushroom bisque

Free of EGG SOY NUT SUGAR OIL

SERVES 6

The rich aromas of this bisque will fill your senses with the earth and woods after a rain. Adding a pinch of cardamom in combination with the nutmeg is an effective way to draw out the soup's essence. Its deep, full-bodied flavor and color are further intensified by the fusion of fresh and dried mushrooms.

½ ounce dried porcini mushrooms

¾ cup hot water

1 pound fresh button mushrooms, sliced

1 pound fresh portobello mushrooms

1 cup dry white wine

1 large yellow onion, coarsely chopped

4 cups Chicken Stock (page 176) or Vegetable Stock (page 177)

2 medium russet potatoes, peeled and cut into 2-inch pieces

¼ cup chopped flat-leaf parsley

½ teaspoon salt

¼ teaspoon freshly ground black pepper

¼ teaspoon ground nutmeg

Pinch ground cardamom

1 cup Dairy Milk Alternative (page 173), plus more if needed

Parsley sprigs, for garnish (optional)

TO RECONSTITUTE THE PORCINIS: Place the porcinis in a small bowl with the hot water. Allow them to soak for 20 minutes, swishing occasionally to loosen any grit. Lift the mushrooms out of the water with a slotted spoon. Using a fine-mesh sieve, strain the liquid over a bowl to remove any sediment. Reserve the liquid and set aside.

TO PREPARE THE PORTOBELLOS: Gently twist off the stems. Then lightly scrape out the black gills and discard. Slice the mushrooms in half and thinly slice the caps.

TO MAKE THE SOUP: In a large saucepan over medium-high heat, combine all the mushrooms with ½ cup of the wine. Steam-sauté, stirring frequently, until all the liquid has evaporated and the mushrooms are lightly browned, 12 to 15 minutes. Set aside ½ cup of the mushrooms. To the remaining mushrooms, add the onion and the remaining ½ cup of wine. Continue sautéing until the liquid is fully absorbed and the onions are softened, 3 to 5 minutes.

Add the stock, reserved mushroom liquid, potatoes, parsley, salt, pepper, nutmeg, and cardamom to the onion mixture. Bring to a boil; cover, decrease the heat to low, and simmer until the potatoes are tender when pierced with a fork, about 25 minutes.

Remove the soup from the heat and ladle half of it into a blender, along with ½ cup of the milk. Cover and puree until smooth, about 1 minute. Empty the blender and repeat with the remaining soup and the remaining ½ cup of milk. Transfer the pureed soup back to the saucepan, add the reserved mushrooms, and stir. Thin the soup, if necessary, by adding a little more milk, ¼ cup at a time, until the desired consistency is achieved. Taste and correct the seasonings. Reheat over low heat, stirring occasionally, until heated through, taking care not to boil the soup. Ladle the soup into bowls and garnish with parsley sprigs.

spinach lentil soup

Free of EGG SOY NUT SUGAR OIL

SERVES 6

When I was growing up lentil soup was a staple in our home. I've expanded on this favorite by adding kombu, a sea vegetable that helps with the digestibility of legumes, while adding a good dose of minerals into the broth.

1 large yellow onion, finely chopped

4 carrots, peeled, cut into ½-inch dice

2 stalks celery, cut into ½-inch dice

¼ cup dry-packed sun-dried tomatoes, cut into ¼-inch pieces

2 cloves garlic, minced

4 cups water

4 cups Vegetable Stock (page 177) or Chicken Stock (page 176)

1¼ cups uncooked brown lentils

2 strips kombu, about 2 by 4 inches (optional)

½ teaspoon freshly ground black pepper

3 cups fresh spinach leaves, tightly packed, coarsely chopped

TO PREPARE THE SOUP: Heat a large saucepan over medium-high heat. Add the onion and 2 tablespoons of water, stirring frequently, until the onion is tender, about 3 minutes. Add the garlic and sauté 1 minute longer. Add the carrots, celery, sun-dried tomatoes, water, stock, lentils, kombu, and pepper. Bring to a boil. Cover and decrease the heat to low. Simmer until the lentils are just tender, about 35 minutes. Remove the kombu and transfer it to a cutting board. Mince the kombu and return it to the pot. Add the spinach and continue cooking for 3 minutes, stirring occasionally until the spinach has wilted. Ladle the soup into bowls and serve.

cabbage bisque

Free of EGG SOY NUT SUGAR OIL

SERVES 6

This delicious, nourishing soup has a delightful, silky smooth texture. By first blanching the cabbage, you remove any bitterness.

1¹/₂ **pounds green cabbage, halved and cored**

1 **large yellow onion, coarsely chopped**

2 **tablespoons dry white wine**

2¹/₃ **cups Chicken Stock (page 176) or Vegetable Stock (page 177)**

1¹/₂ **pounds russet potatoes, peeled and coarsely chopped**

1 **teaspoon minced fresh dill, or** ¹/₂ **teaspoon dried**

¹/₄ **cup chopped fresh parsley**

³/₄ **teaspoon salt**

¹/₈ **teaspoon ground white pepper**

2 **cups Dairy Milk Alternative (page 173), plus more if needed**

TO PREPARE THE CABBAGE: Set cabbage in a large bowl and pour enough boiling water over it to cover completely. Let the cabbage stand until it has softened, about 8 minutes. Transfer the cabbage to a colander and drain well, about 20 minutes. Slice the drained cabbage into strips about 2 inches long. Reserve 2 cups of the sliced cabbage in a small bowl, and set aside.

TO MAKE THE SOUP: Heat a large saucepan over medium-high heat. Add the onion and wine, stirring frequently, until the onion is tender, about 3 minutes. Add the cabbage, stock, potatoes, dill, parsley, salt, and pepper. Bring to a boil, cover, decrease the heat to low, and simmer until the vegetables are tender, about 25 minutes.

TO PUREE THE SOUP: Remove the soup from the heat and ladle half of it into a blender, along with 1 cup of the milk. Cover and puree until smooth, about 1 minute. Empty the blender into a bowl and repeat with the remaining soup and remaining 1 cup of milk. Transfer the pureed soup back into the saucepan and add the reserved 2 cups of cabbage, stirring to incorporate. Thin the soup if necessary by adding a little more milk, ¹/₄ cup at a time, until the desired consistency is achieved. Taste and correct the seasoning. Reheat over low heat, stirring occasionally, until heated through, taking care not to boil the soup.

chilled summer chowder

Free of EGG SOY* NUT SUGAR OIL

SERVES 6

Inspired by my summer garden, this soup is fresh, light, and ultra refreshing on a hot summer day. Any combination of chopped vegetables will work here, so use your imagination and create your own signature toppings.

SOUP

4 medium English cucumbers, peeled and chopped

2¹/₂ cups plain dairy-free yogurt*

1 teaspoon freshly squeezed lime juice

¹/₂ teaspoon sea salt

¹/₂ teaspoon white pepper

TOPPING

¹/₂ cup seeded and chopped vine-ripened red tomato

¹/₂ cup seeded and chopped vine-ripened yellow tomato

¹/₂ cup chopped zucchini

¹/₂ cup seeded and chopped orange bell pepper

¹/₄ cup chopped fennel

¹/₄ cup chopped green onions

1¹/₂ tablespoons apple cider vinegar

1¹/₂ teaspoons Date Syrup (page 189) or honey

2 tablespoons minced fresh basil or mint leaves, for garnish

TO PREPARE THE SOUP: Combine the cucumbers, yogurt, lime, salt, and pepper in a blender. Cover and puree until smooth and creamy, about 2 minutes. Transfer to a glass container, cover and chill in the refrigerator for 2 hours. Meanwhile, in a large bowl, combine the tomatoes, zucchini, bell pepper, fennel, and onion. In a small bowl, combine the apple cider vinegar and date syrup, whisking to blend. Pour the vinegar over the vegetable mixture and gently toss to combine. Cover and chill for 2 hours before serving.

TO SERVE THE SOUP: Ladle the soup into shallow bowls and top with about ¹/₃ cup of the topping in the center of the bowl. Sprinkle with minced basil.

salmon *and* white corn chowder

Free of EGG SOY NUT SUGAR OIL

SERVES 6

Delicately flavored with a slight sweetness from the corn, this chowder is rich in texture and taste. Poaching the salmon with the skin on releases just enough oil to enrich the broth.

3 (8-ounce) bottles clam juice

¼ cup dry white wine

1 (16-ounce) salmon fillet with skin

3 medium leeks, white and pale green parts only, thinly sliced

1¼ pounds white potatoes, peeled and cut into ½-inch pieces

2 tablespoon Gluten-Free Flour Mix (page 172)

2½ cups Dairy Milk Alternative (page 173), plus more if needed

1 cup white corn kernels, fresh (about 2 ears) or frozen

¼ teaspoon salt

¼ teaspoon freshly ground black pepper

2 tablespoons minced green onion, green parts only, for garnish

TO PREPARE THE SALMON: Bring the clam juice and wine to a boil in a saucepan over medium-high heat. Decrease the heat to low and add the salmon. Cover and simmer until cooked through,

8 to 10 minutes. With a slotted spoon, transfer the salmon to a plate and allow to cool, reserving the clam juice. With a fork, flake the salmon into small pieces, discarding the skin and bones. Set aside.

TO ASSEMBLE THE SOUP: Heat a large saucepan over medium-high heat and add the leeks, stirring frequently, until soft. As the leeks begin to caramelize, add 2 tablespoons of the reserved clam juice to keep them from sticking to the pan, about 4 minutes. Add the remaining reserved clam juice and the potatoes and bring to a boil. Decrease the heat to low, cover, and simmer until the potatoes are tender, about 10 minutes.

Meanwhile, in a blender combine the milk and flour, cover, and whirl at top speed for about 30 seconds to blend. Pour the mixture into a saucepan and cook over medium-high heat, whisking constantly until the sauce begins to thicken, about 3 minutes.

Add the milk mixture to the potato mixture and bring to a simmer over low heat. Stir in the salmon, corn, salt, and pepper, and cook over low heat until heated through, taking care not to boil the soup. Taste and correct the seasonings. Ladle the soup into bowls and garnish with green onions.

the **dairy-free** and **gluten-free** kitchen

fish and shellfish

Seafood is enjoyed around the world and you'll find a pretty good selection in most supermarkets. That's great news for the adventurous chef looking to try new recipes, but can sometimes play havoc on ecosystems when overfishing and pollution are unchecked. For that reason I recommend looking for wild-caught and farmed seafood that has been sourced from fisheries that practice sustainable harvesting. It's healthy for you and the oceans. For current sustainability seafood guides, please see the Resources (page 191) for more information.

poached cod over glass noodles

Free of EGG NUT SUGAR OIL

SERVES 4

This dish is a restaurant-quality entrée that is both beautiful and simple to assemble. If you can't find fresh cod, then substitute another type of white fish, such as haddock, turbot, or flounder.

---

4 (4-ounce) ling cod fillets

2 tablespoons gluten-free tamari

4 cups Chicken Stock (page 176)

$1/4$ cup Date Syrup (page 189) or honey

$1/2$ cup Chopped Tomatoes (page 179)

2 tablespoons apple cider vinegar

3 tablespoons peeled, minced fresh ginger

3 cloves garlic, thinly sliced

1 stalk lemongrass, bottom half cut into thirds and lightly crushed

$1/4$ teaspoon hot pepper sauce, or to taste

2 ounces dried bean thread noodles

4 small baby bok choy

$1/4$ cup chopped fresh cilantro, for garnish

$1/4$ cup thinly sliced green onion, white and green parts, for garnish

---

Place the fish on a plate and drizzle with tamari, coating both sides, and set aside.

TO PREPARE THE FISH: In a large 12-inch sauté pan, combine the stock, date syrup, tomatoes, vinegar, ginger, garlic, lemongrass, and hot pepper sauce, stirring to blend. Bring the mixture to a boil, reduce the heat to medium-low, and simmer for about 12 minutes, stirring occasionally. Meanwhile, soak the noodles in a bowl of warm water to cover, and set aside. Transfer the fish to the sauté pan of poaching liquid and arrange the bok choy on top; cover, and simmer until the fish is almost opaque, 6 to 8 minutes.

TO ASSEMBLE THE DISH: In a colander, drain the noodles and equally distribute them among four shallow serving bowls. Using a slotted spoon carefully place the filets on top of the noodles and place the bok choy alongside. Bring the poaching liquid to a boil, and boil the mixture uncovered for 3 to 4 minutes. Ladle the liquid equally among the four bowls. Garnish with cilantro and green onions. Serve immediately.

baked salmon *in* parchment

Free of EGG SOY NUT SUGAR OIL

SERVES 4

These festive little packets are an extremely forgiving way to prepare fish. The fish and vegetables cook and steam en papillote, *the French term for "in paper," retaining all their flavor and moisture. This main course creates an elegant presentation, perfect for a special evening or holiday dinner, and the clean-up is a snap.*

4 (4-ounce) boneless fresh salmon fillets, about ³/₄ inch thick

2 carrots, julienned

1 red bell pepper, seeded, ribbed, and julienned

1 leak, white and pale green part only, julienned

2 cloves garlic, thinly sliced

2 tablespoons minced flat-leaf parsley

2 teaspoons freshly squeezed lemon juice

2 tablespoons dry white wine

¹/₄ teaspoon salt

¹/₈ teaspoon freshly ground black pepper

Lemon wedges, for garnish (optional)

Preheat oven to 375°F.

TO PREPARE THE PARCHMENT PAPER: Cut 4 pieces of parchment paper measuring 15 by 36 inches.

Fold them in half like a book and draw a large half heart shape on each. Cut out the heart and open it flat on the counter.

TO ASSEMBLE THE PARCHMENT PACKETS: Evenly distribute the carrots, bell pepper, leek, and parsley on the parchment paper and arrange them in the center and to one side of the fold. Lay the salmon on top of the vegetables and sprinkle with lemon juice, wine, salt, and pepper. Fold the other side of the parchment over the fish. Starting at the top of the heart shape, fold up the edges of the paper, overlapping and crimping the edges tightly as you make your way around the heart. When you reach the tip, twist the paper several times to secure it so that when cooking, the steam will not escape.

TO BAKE THE FISH: Place the parchment packets on a rimmed baking sheet. The packets can be made up to 4 hours ahead and refrigerated. If refrigerated, allow the packets to reach room temperature, about 1 hour, before placing them in the oven. Bake the fish for 20 minutes. Transfer to individual plates and carefully open each packet, allowing the steam to escape before serving. Serve immediately.

mahi mahi *with* white beans *and* sun-dried tomato cream

SERVES 4

If you cook the beans ahead of time or use canned beans, you can assemble this entrée in just minutes. The sauce can be prepared the day before and rewarmed while the fish is cooking. You can use any firm white fish in this recipe, including Pacific halibut or sturgeon and if you prefer, the fish can be grilled.

1 large yellow onion, coarsely chopped

1 cup chopped carrot (about 2 medium)

1 cup chopped celery (about 3 stalks)

3 cloves garlic

$^{1}/_{4}$ cup water

6 fresh sage leaves, chopped

2 sprigs winter savory or thyme

1 bay leaf

1 tablespoon grated lemon zest (2 to 3 lemons)

$^{1}/_{4}$ cup dry white wine

2 cups cooked white beans or great Northern beans (see page 180)

$^{1}/_{2}$ cup Chopped Tomatoes with their juice (page 179)

$^{1}/_{2}$ cup Chicken Stock (page 176)

$^{1}/_{2}$ teaspoon salt

$^{1}/_{4}$ teaspoon freshly ground black pepper

1 tablespoon canola oil

4 (4-ounce) mahi mahi (dorado) steaks, $^{3}/_{4}$ to 1 inch thick

$^{3}/_{4}$ cup Sun-Dried Tomato Cream (page 122)

Lemon wedges, for garnish (optional)

TO PREPARE THE BEANS: Heat a large, heavy saucepan over medium-high heat. Add the onion, carrot, and celery and sauté, stirring constantly, until tender, about 3 minutes. Add the water to the pan and steam-sauté 2 minutes more. Add the garlic, sage, savory, bay leaf, zest, and wine; stir for 1 minute. Add the beans, tomatoes, chicken stock, salt, and pepper and toss to combine all ingredients. Cover and simmer until just heated through, about 15 minutes. Remove from the heat and cover to keep warm.

TO PREPARE THE FISH: Heat the oil in a large skillet over medium-high heat until hot. Lightly salt and pepper the mahi mahi. Place the fish in the hot skillet, partially covering the skillet with a lid to reduce spattering. Cook for 4 to 5 minutes. Flip the fish and continue to cook the other side until lightly browned, 3 to 4 minutes.

To serve, spoon the beans onto the center of each plate and place the mahi mahi on top. Spoon about 2 tablespoons of the Sun-Dried Tomato Cream on top, and serve immediately.

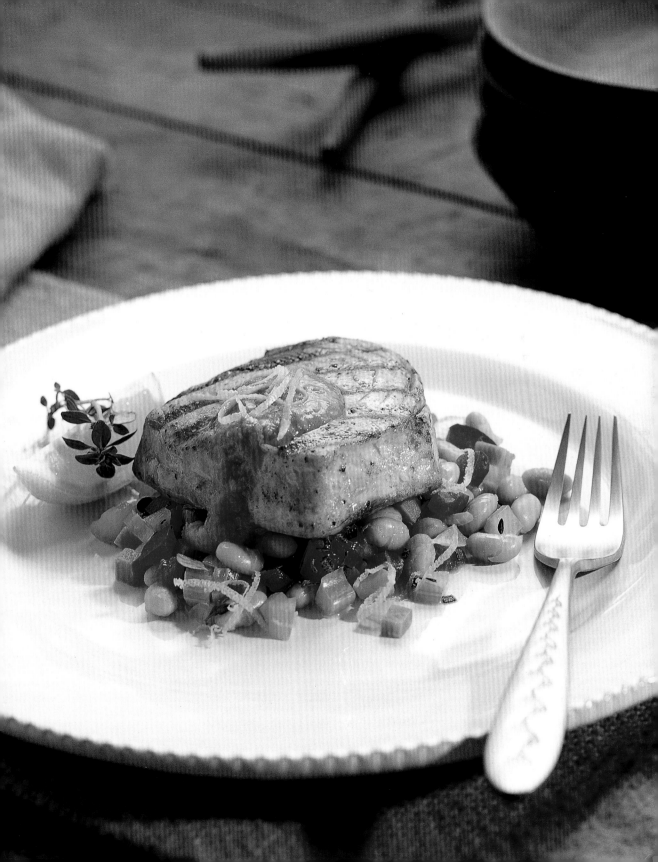

halibut *in* swiss chard wraps

Free of EGG SOY NUT SUGAR

SERVES 4

These tasty little packages make a nice presentation for a special weekend dinner with family and friends. If you prefer, substitute New Zealand cod (hoki) or striped bass for the halibut.

FILLING

1 (8-ounce) bottle clam juice

1$\frac{1}{2}$ ounces dry-packed sun-dried tomatoes (about $\frac{3}{4}$ cup)

4 cloves garlic, minced

2 tablespoons olive oil

$\frac{1}{4}$ teaspoon dried lemongrass

$\frac{1}{2}$ teaspoon salt

$\frac{1}{4}$ teaspoon freshly ground black pepper

WRAPS

8 large Swiss chard leaves, thick stems removed

4 (4-ounce) skinless, boneless fresh halibut fillets, about 1$\frac{1}{2}$ inches thick and 2 inches wide

SAUCE

$\frac{1}{3}$ cup Dairy Milk Alternative (page 173)

$\frac{1}{4}$ cup dry sherry

1 tablespoon freshly squeezed lemon juice

1 tablespoon Gluten-Free Flour Mix (page 172)

4 thin slices lemon, for garnish (optional)

TO PREPARE THE FILLING: Combine the clam juice and tomatoes in a small covered saucepan over medium-high heat, bring to a boil, and boil for 2 minutes. Remove the saucepan from the heat and allow it to sit, covered, for 15 minutes.

With a slotted spoon, transfer the tomatoes to a cutting board and mince. Reserve the clam juice. Combine the tomatoes, garlic, olive oil, lemongrass, salt, and pepper in a bowl, and stir to blend.

TO PREPARE THE CHARD: Place a large pot of water fitted with a steaming basket over medium-high heat and bring to a boil. Place the chard in the basket and steam until just wilted, about 30 seconds. Remove from the basket and rinse the chard under cold running water; drain well and pat dry.

Place 2 chard leaves together, overlapping the long sides. Place one fish fillet crosswise over the leaves near the stem end. Spoon 1 tablespoon of the tomato mixture over the fillet and spread evenly. Fold the chard over the fish and roll up. Repeat with the remaining chard and fish. Place the wraps seam-side down in an 8 by 11 by 2-inch baking dish.

TO PREPARE THE SAUCE: Preheat the oven to 350°F. In a blender combine the reserved clam juice, milk, sherry, lemon juice, and flour. Cover and whirl at top speed for about 30 seconds. Pour the mixture into a saucepan and cook over medium-high heat, whisking constantly, until the sauce begins to thicken, 3 to 4 minutes. (The sauce will be thick but will thin while baking.) Pour the sauce over the wraps, cover with aluminum foil, and bake for 40 minutes. Spoon the sauce from the baking dish onto each plate and place a wrap on top of the sauce. Garnish each wrap with a slice of lemon.

shrimp tacos

Free of EGG SOY NUT SUGAR OIL

SERVES 4

Serve these tacos family-style by setting out all of the toppings in advance.

TOPPINGS

Chunky Guacamole (page 126)

Pico De Gallo (page 126)

1 cup shredded lettuce

1/2 bunch fresh cilantro

4 lime wedges

FILLING

2 teaspoons chili powder

1 cup shredded lettuce

1/2 teaspoon ground cumin

1/2 teaspoon onion powder

1/2 teaspoon garlic powder

1/4 teaspoon salt

1/4 cup water

2 tablespoons freshly squeezed lime juice

16 large shrimp, tails and shells removed

16 corn tortillas

Place the toppings in separate bowls and set aside. To warm the tortillas wrap them in a damp dish towel and steam in the microwave for 30 seconds, or warm in a skillet for 2 minutes.

TO PREPARE THE FILLING: In a small bowl combine the chili powder, cumin, onion powder, garlic powder, and salt, stirring to blend. In a large skillet over medium-high heat add the spice mixture and cook until fragrant, stirring constantly, about 1 minute. Add the water, lime juice, and shrimp, stirring to blend. Cook the shrimp until opaque in the center, 2 to 3 minutes. Avoid overcooking or they will become tough. Transfer to a bowl and serve with tortillas and toppings.

pecan-crusted trout

Free of SOY SUGAR

SERVES 4

The rich and crunchy texture of the pecans pro-vides a nice contrast to the light and flaky trout, resulting in fish that is crisp on the outside and moist inside. To give this recipe a southern flair, add more cayenne pepper and use farmed catfish in place of the trout.

1 cup Gluten-Free Bread Crumbs (page 185)

$^1/_2$ cup finely chopped pecans

$^1/_2$ teaspoon salt

$^1/_2$ teaspoon chili powder

$^1/_4$ teaspoon cayenne pepper

1 tablespoon olive oil

2 cloves garlic, minced

4 (10- to 12-ounce) whole trout, butterflied and boned, with skin

2 tablespoons canola oil, for pan frying

Lemon wedges, for garnish (optional)

Preheat the oven to 400°F.

TO PREPARE THE FISH: Combine the bread crumbs, pecans, salt, chili powder, and cayenne in a small bowl and stir to blend. Heat the olive oil in a small saucepan over medium heat. Add the garlic and sauté for 1 minute. Open the trout and place them skin-side down on a large baking sheet; brush with the garlic oil. Coat the trout with the nut mixture, pressing it to help it adhere.

Heat 1 tablespoon of the canola oil in a large, nonstick skillet over medium-high heat until hot. Place 2 trout, coated-side down, into the hot skillet, and cook for about 2 minutes. Using a spatula, flip the trout and transfer to the baking sheet, coated-side up. Repeat with the remaining 1 tablespoon of the oil. Bake the trout, uncovered, until just opaque in the center, 4 to 5 minutes.

Transfer the fish to individual plates and garnish with lemon wedges. Serve immediately.

roasted hot *and* spicy crab

SERVES 6

I love to serve this crab for dinner on New Year's Eve, when lingering over a meal is a treat. Serve it in front of a crackling fire with a tossed green salad and plenty of champagne. Spices often contain hidden sources of gluten so be sure to check that the chili powder and hot pepper sauce you're using are both gluten-free.

¼ cup olive oil

3 tablespoons minced garlic (6 to 9 cloves)

2 tablespoons peeled, minced fresh ginger

2 tablespoons minced red onion

3 tablespoons freshly squeezed lemon juice (1 to 2 lemons)

2 teaspoons chili powder

1 tablespoon hot pepper sauce

1 teaspoon sugar

¼ teaspoon crushed red pepper flakes, more or less to taste

5 Dungeness crabs, cooked, cleaned, and cracked (about 6 pounds total)

Lemon wedges, for garnish (optional)

TO MAKE THE MARINADE: Heat the olive oil in a large saucepan over medium-high heat. Sauté the garlic, ginger, and onion for about 1 minute. Add the lemon juice, chili powder, hot pepper sauce, sugar, and pepper flakes, and stir until the marinade is well blended and the sugar has dissolved, about 2 minutes. Remove the saucepan from the heat and allow the mixture to cool slightly, about 5 minutes.

TO MARINATE THE CRAB: Place the crab in a large bowl or heavy resealable plastic bag, pour the marinade over the crab, and toss to coat thoroughly. Cover and refrigerate for 1 to 3 hours, turning the crab occasionally.

TO ROAST THE CRAB: Preheat the oven to 500°F. Transfer the crab and marinade to a heavy, 12 by 16-inch roasting pan. Roast the crab, uncovered, until the garlic is golden brown and the crab is hot, 10 to 15 minutes. Arrange the crab on a platter and garnish with lemon wedges.

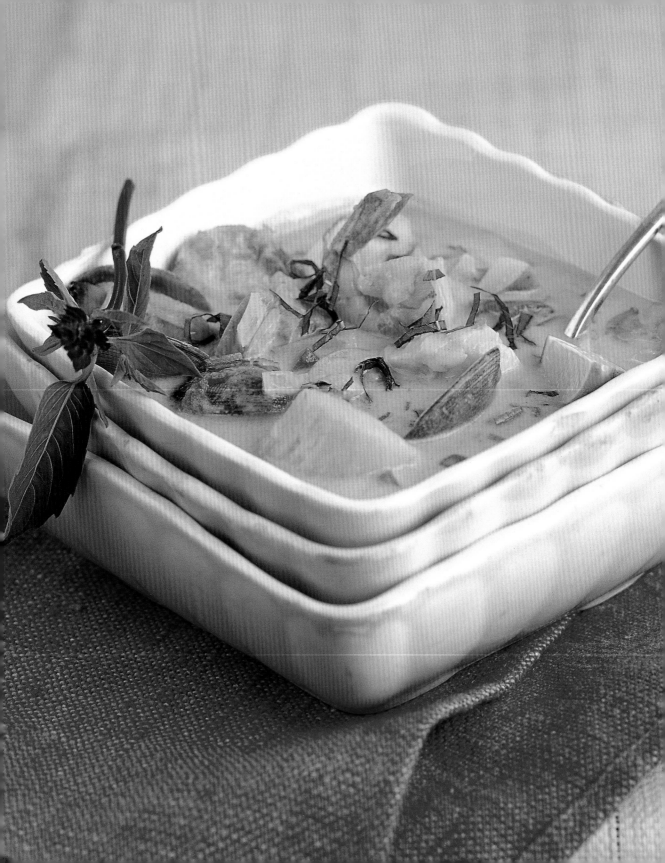

coconut-lime seafood stew

Free of EGG SOY SUGAR OIL

SERVES 4

Without question, this was my father's favorite dish. And no wonder—it's loaded with fresh seafood, has a rich and creamy broth, and is altogether deeply satisfying. The turmeric gives the broth a lovely golden hue with lemon undertones and makes the dish shine.

When you purchase live mollusks (shellfish) from the market, it is important to remove them from the plastic bag as soon as you get home. Store them in the refrigerator in a bowl with about 1/4 inch of water and a wet paper towel draped over the top of the bowl. This ensures freshness until you are ready to use them.

1 large yellow onion, chopped

1 tablespoon peeled, minced fresh ginger

1 teaspoon ground turmeric

1 (8-ounce) bottle clam juice

3/4 cup water

2 cups Chopped Tomatoes with their juice (page 179)

1 3/4 pounds new red potatoes, cut into 1-inch pieces

1 teaspoon grated lime zest

1/2 teaspoon salt

1/4 teaspoon freshly ground black pepper

1 cup whole fresh basil leaves, tightly packed

1 pound fresh littleneck clams or mussels, scrubbed

1 (14-ounce) can unsweetened coconut milk

1/2 pound fresh skinless, boneless halibut steak, cut into 1-inch cubes

1/2 pound fresh jumbo prawns, deveined

1/2 pound fresh jumbo scallops

2 tablespoons freshly squeezed lime juice (1 to 2 limes)

Lime wedges, for garnish (optional)

TO PREPARE THE STEW: Heat a large, heavy saucepan over medium-high heat. Add the onion and sauté, stirring constantly, until tender, about 2 minutes. Add 1/4 cup of the water to the pan and steam-sauté 2 minutes more. Stir in the ginger and turmeric until blended, about 1 minute. Stir in the clam juice, 1/4 cup of the water, tomatoes, potatoes, lime zest, salt, and pepper. Bring to a boil; cover, decrease the heat to low, and simmer for 18 to 20 minutes, stirring occasionally. Add the basil and clams and continue simmering until the clams open, 5 to 7 minutes. Discard any that do not open. Add the coconut milk, halibut, prawns, scallops, and lime juice, and stir until incorporated. Cover and simmer until just heated through, 3 to 4 minutes. Taste and correct the seasonings. Ladle into bowls, garnish each with a lime wedge, and serve immediately.

asian linguine and clams

Free of   EGG   NUT   SUGAR

SERVES 4

Ingredients such as ginger, sesame oil, cilantro, and tamari add an Asian spin to classic linguine and clams, making this dish an aromatic delight for the senses. Be sure to use fresh ginger, as dried will not offer the desired flavor in this recipe. Jalapeño peppers can vary in heat, from medium to very hot. Be sure you taste before adding it to the dish.

1 (16-ounce) package gluten-free linguine or spaghetti noodles

3 tablespoons toasted sesame oil

1 large yellow onion, finely chopped

1 red bell pepper, seeded, ribbed, and julienned

1 1/2 tablespoons peeled, minced fresh ginger

2 cloves garlic, minced

1 seeded, minced jalapeño pepper, more or less to taste

1 (8-ounce) bottle clam juice

1/2 cup plus 2 tablespoons water

3 tablespoons rice vinegar

3 tablespoons sake

2 tablespoons gluten-free tamari

32 fresh littleneck clams, scrubbed

1/4 cup thinly sliced green onion, white and green parts

1/4 cup chopped fresh cilantro

TO PREPARE THE PASTA: Bring 3 quarts of water to a boil in a large saucepan over high heat. Add the linguine to the water, bring to a boil, and stir. Cook the linguine, uncovered, according to the package directions, taking care not to overcook it. Drain the linguine in a colander and allow it to cool slightly. Transfer to a large bowl and toss with 1 tablespoon of the sesame oil to coat.

In the same large saucepan, heat 2 tablespoons of water over medium-high heat. Add the onion, bell pepper, ginger, garlic, and jalapeño, stirring frequently, until they begin to soften, about 5 minutes. Add the clam juice, the remaining 1/2 cup of water, vinegar, sake, and tamari. Bring to a boil and add the clams. Cover and cook until the clams open, 5 to 7 minutes, discarding any that do not open. Toss with the remaining 2 tablespoons of the sesame oil. Taste and correct the seasonings. Spoon the clams and sauce over the pasta, sprinkle with green onion and cilantro, and serve.

poultry and meat

Choose animals raised by local farmers committed to high animal welfare standards. Grass-fed, pasture-raised beef is a great example of how much the way an animal is raised will affect the quality of the meat it produces. When a cow is treated with respect and given access to a natural diet, it will be leaner, have more healthful omega-3s, and a nice, bold flavor. Further, deciding to eat smaller, more healthful portions of meat benefits the environment, our families, local communities—and the animals.

chicken vera cruz

Free of EGG SOY NUT SUGAR OIL

SERVES 4

The flavors of this Latin-inspired entrée are fresh, warm, and inviting. It has several parts—the black bean sauce, succulent chicken, and luscious avocado, all crowned with a zesty salsa. Begin by making the black bean sauce, then continue with the other elements. If you cook, shock, and refrigerate the black beans the day before, the sauce will take minutes to assemble. Just remember to save the cooking liquid from the beans—you'll need it to make the sauce.

1 teaspoon garlic powder

$1/2$ teaspoon salt

$1/2$ teaspoon freshly ground black pepper

$1/8$ teaspoon ground cumin

4 boneless, skinless chicken breast halves, lightly pounded

1 cup Black Bean Sauce (page 121)

2 ripe avocados, halved

Pico de Gallo (page 126)

TO PREPARE THE CHICKEN: Preheat the grill to 350°F (a medium-hot fire). In a small bowl, combine the garlic powder, salt, pepper, and cumin; stir to blend. Lightly sprinkle both sides of the chicken with the seasonings. Place the chicken on the hot grill and grill for 2 to 3 minutes, rotate the chicken once 45 degrees to make cross-hatched grill marks, then grill for 2 minutes longer. Turn the chicken over and repeat until it is cooked through and the juices run clear, a total of 8 to 10 minutes cooking time.

TO ASSEMBLE THE DISH: Spoon about $1/4$ cup of the black bean sauce into the center of 4 shallow bowls or rimmed plates. Place a chicken breast in the center of each pool of sauce. Slice each avocado half into 5 equal pieces and fan them out on top of the chicken. Top with Pico de Gallo, and serve.

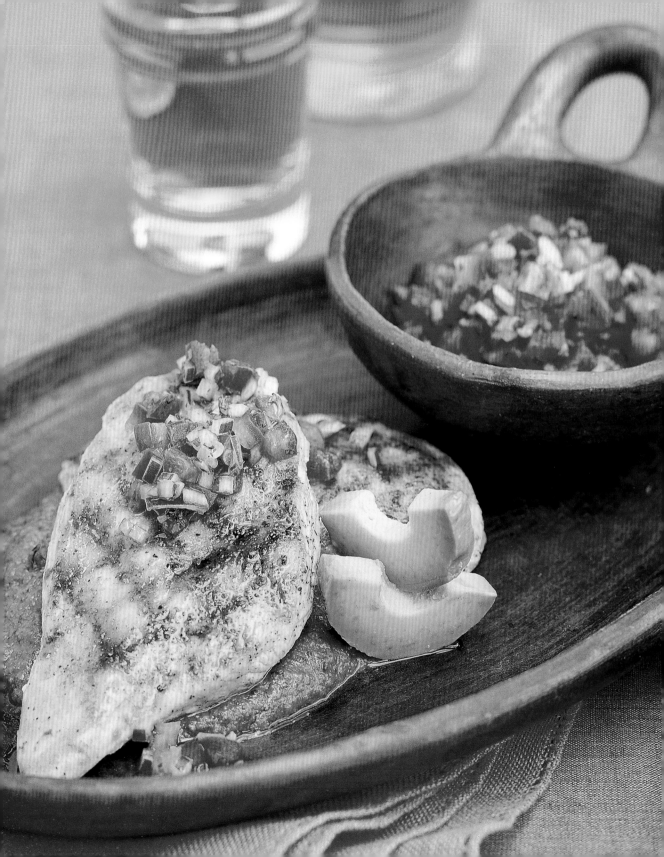

chicken *with* potato *and* leek *in* tarragon cream

Free of EGG SOY NUT SUGAR

SERVES 4

This French-inspired dish is quick to assemble and can easily be made a day ahead; just cover and refrigerate. If refrigerated, allow an additional 10 minutes of baking time. For a boost of calcium, serve it alongside your favorite steamed or sautéed dark greens, such as kale, broccolini, or collard greens.

1 tablespoon olive oil

4 boneless, skinless chicken breast halves, pounded to a $1/4$-inch thickness

$1/2$ teaspoon salt

$1/4$ teaspoon freshly ground black pepper

2 cloves garlic, minced

2 medium Yukon Gold potatoes, unpeeled, sliced $1/8$ inch thick or less

2 large leeks, white and light green part only, julienned

12 slices lemon, cut $1/8$ inch thick or less (1 to 2 lemons)

1 cup Chicken Stock (page 176)

$1/3$ cup dry white wine

$1 1/2$ cups Dairy Milk Alternative (page 173)

1 tablespoon freshly squeezed lemon juice

2 tablespoons Gluten-Free Flour Mix (page 172)

$1/4$ cup minced fresh tarragon

Tarragon sprigs, for garnish (optional)

TO PREPARE THE CHICKEN: Preheat the oven to 350°F. Heat the olive oil in a large skillet over medium-high heat. Lightly season the chicken with salt and pepper. Place the chicken in the hot skillet and sear each side until just browned, about 2 minutes.

Remove the chicken from the skillet and place side by side in an 8 by 11 by 2-inch glass baking dish. Sprinkle the chicken with the garlic and fan about 5 slices of potato on top of each chicken breast. Next, evenly arrange the leeks on top of the potatoes, and finish by fanning about 3 slices of lemon on top of the leeks. Set aside.

TO PREPARE THE SAUCE: In a blender combine the chicken stock, wine, milk, lemon juice, and flour. Cover the blender and whirl at top speed for about 30 seconds to blend. Pour the mixture into a saucepan, add the tarragon, and cook over medium-high heat, whisking constantly, until the sauce begins to thicken, about 3 minutes. Taste and correct the seasonings.

TO BAKE AND SERVE THE CHICKEN: Pour the sauce slowly over the layered chicken. Cover with foil and bake until the sauce is bubbly, about 40 minutes. Remove the dish from the oven and let it stand, covered, for 5 minutes. Serve with remaining sauce and a tarragon sprig garnish.

mediterranean roast chicken

Free of EGG SOY NUT SUGAR

SERVES 4

Whether I am preparing a hearty meal for my family or for a casual get-together with friends, succulent roast chicken is a staple in our home. For a classic family-style meal, pair the chicken with Yam and Potato Mashers (page 110) and Roasted Vegetable Medley (page 117). For a more formal dinner party serve the chicken with Corn Soufflé (page 102); either way it's delicious.

There are countless ways to roast a chicken but this method is my favorite. Elevating the chicken on a rack in the roasting pan permits the heat to circulate around the chicken and guarantees a uniform, crispy, golden brown skin. To keep the bird moist, let it rest uncovered before carving. This allows the juices to draw back into the meat instead of draining out when cut.

1 (3½- to 6-pound) fresh whole roasting chicken, giblets removed

½ medium yellow onion, quartered

2 tablespoons minced fresh rosemary

1 tablespoon olive oil

2 teaspoons minced fresh oregano

1 teaspoon minced fresh thyme

½ teaspoon garlic powder

½ teaspoon coarse salt

¼ teaspoon coarsely ground black pepper

TO PREPARE THE CHICKEN: Rinse the chicken inside and out and pat dry with paper towels. Place the chicken on a rack in the roasting pan and set aside. Position the oven rack in the bottom third of the oven and preheat the oven to 375°F.

TO PREPARE THE RUB: Combine the rosemary, olive oil, oregano, thyme, garlic powder, salt, and pepper in a small bowl and mix to blend. Starting at the neck end, loosen the skin around the breast meat by sliding your hand under the skin. Using your hand, spread 2 teaspoons of the herb mixture under the skin of the chicken, evenly covering the breast meat. Rub the remaining herb mixture over the outside skin of the chicken and in the main cavity. Place the onion inside the main cavity and tuck the wing tips under the chicken.

TO COOK THE CHICKEN: Roast the chicken for 1½ to 2 hours, depending on the size of the bird, or until an instant-read thermometer inserted into the thickest part of the thigh, without touching the bone, registers 165°F. Remove the pan from the oven and allow the chicken to rest for about 10 minutes before carving.

chicken *in* mushroom sauce

Free of EGG SOY NUT SUGAR

SERVES 4

*Basic as this dish is, it always gets rave reviews
whether I am serving it for my family or for a large
group. Once the dish is assembled, it can be kept
warm in the oven, all the while continuing to baste
itself in the mushroom sauce. My family prefers
dark meat to white so I use chicken thighs but this
recipe is equally suited to boneless, skinless breast
halves; just be sure to pound them to an equal
thickness of about $1/4$ inch.*

$1^1/_2$ **pounds boneless skinless chicken thighs,
trimmed**

$1/_2$ **teaspoon salt**

$1/_4$ **teaspoon freshly ground black pepper**

$1/_4$ **cup Gluten-Free Flour Mix (page 172)**

2 tablespoons olive oil

1 large yellow onion, halved and thinly sliced

2 cloves garlic, minced

1 pound white mushrooms, thinly sliced

$1/_2$ **cup Marsala wine**

$1/_4$ **cup dry cooking sherry**

1 cup Chicken Stock (page 176)

6 thyme sprigs

$1/_4$ **cup minced flat-leaf parsley**

Yam and Potato Mashers (page 110)

**Braised Greens with Caramelized Onion
(page 114)**

TO PREPARE THE CHICKEN: Sprinkle the chicken with
salt and pepper. Place the flour on a plate and
dust both sides of the chicken with the flour,
shaking off any excess. In a large sauté pan heat
the olive oil over medium-high heat. Add the
chicken and sauté until just brown, turning once,
about 5 minutes each side. Transfer the chicken
to a plate. Add the onion and 2 tablespoons of the
stock to the pan and steam-sauté the onion, stirring frequently, until the onion is tender, about
3 minutes. Add the garlic and sauté 1 minute
longer. Add the mushrooms and cook, stirring
frequently, until the mushrooms are reduced by
half in volume, about 8 minutes. Add the wine,
sherry, and stock to deglaze the pan, scraping up
any brown bits and incorporating them into the
sauce. Add the thyme and bring the sauce to a
boil for about 3 minutes. Return the chicken and
any of its juices to the pan and spoon some of
the mushroom mixture on top. Cover, decrease
the heat to low, and simmer until the chicken is
cooked through and tender, about 30 minutes.

TO SERVE: Place a scoop of the mashed potatoes in
the center of a shallow bowl or dinner plate, and
top with a piece of chicken, spoon the mushroom sauce over the chicken, and garnish with
a sprinkling of parsley. Serve with the braised
greens.

curried stuffed zucchini

SERVES 4

My summertime garden inspired this recipe, when the small zucchini seed I planted in the spring produced an abundance of squash.

STUFFING

1½ **pounds zucchini (4 medium to large)**

1 **tablespoon olive oil**

1 **large yellow onion, finely chopped**

½ **pound ground turkey or 1 (8-ounce) package tempeh, crumbled**

3 **cloves garlic, minced**

1 **red bell pepper, seeded, ribbed, and finely chopped**

½ **cup finely chopped fresh cilantro (about 1 bunch)**

¼ **cup dried currants**

1 **tablespoon fresh lemon juice**

SAUCE

½ **cup Dairy Milk Alternative (page 173)**

1 **tablespoon yellow curry powder**

¼ **teaspoon salt**

¼ **teaspoon freshly ground black pepper**

4 **cups cooked millet**

Lemon slices, for garnish (optional)

TO PREPARE THE ZUCCHINI: Preheat the oven to 350°F. Trim the ends and slice the zucchini in half lengthwise. Using a spoon, core each zucchini, leaving a ½-inch-thick shell. Save the removed pulp, chop, and set aside.

TO PREPARE THE STUFFING: Heat the olive oil in a large skillet over medium-high heat and sauté the onion until soft, about 3 minutes. Add the turkey and garlic, and sauté until evenly browned, about 5 minutes. Add the bell pepper, cilantro, zucchini pulp, currants, and lemon juice. Cover and simmer for 2 to 3 minutes, stirring occasionally. Remove the skillet from the heat and set aside.

Place the zucchini shells in a shallow baking dish, cut-side up. Using a slotted spoon, fill each zucchini shell with the stuffing, reserving the liquid in the skillet.

TO PREPARE THE SAUCE: Place the skillet with the reserved liquid over medium-high heat and bring to a boil. Decrease the heat to low and whisk in the milk, curry powder, salt, and pepper. Whisking constantly, simmer until the curry powder has completely dissolved, 2 to 3 minutes. Spoon over the zucchini and cover with foil. Bake until tender, 25 to 30 minutes.

Divide the millet and zucchini halves among 4 plates. Spoon the sauce over the top. Garnish with a slice of lemon, and serve.

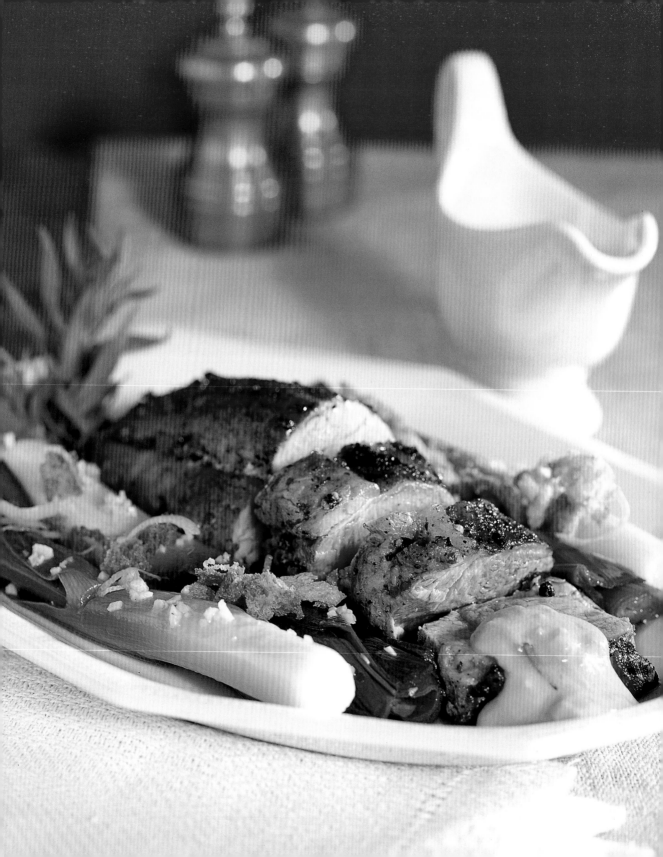

peppered pork tenderloin
in mustard cream sauce

SERVES 6

The searing process used in this recipe produces a delightful crusty pork tenderloin with a subtle infusion of pepper. Mixed peppercorns—red, green, white, and black—can be found in the spice section of your local supermarket. Serve the pork alongside Scalloped Potatoes (page 109) and Lemon-Garlic Crusted Leeks (page 115).

3 tablespoons mixed peppercorns

2 pork tenderloins, trimmed (about 2 pounds total)

½ teaspoon salt

2 tablespoons canola oil

Mustard Cream Sauce (page 124)

TO PREPARE THE PORK: Coarsely grind the peppercorns in a blender or spice grinder. Lightly sprinkle the pork with salt. Press the pepper onto the pork, coating it completely. Heat the oil in a large sauté pan over medium-high heat until hot. Place the pork tenderloins in the hot skillet, partially covering the skillet with a lid to reduce spattering. Brown the pork on all sides and cook until an instant-read meat thermometer inserted into the thickest portion of the meat registers 150°F, 15 to 20 minutes.

TO SERVE THE PORK: Transfer the pork to a cutting board and allow it to rest for 5 minutes. The temperature will continue to rise as it rests. Cut the pork into 1-inch-thick slices. Spoon the sauce onto individual plates and top with the pork.

shepherd's pie

Free of EGG SOY NUT SUGAR

SERVES 4 TO 6

Shepherd's pie can just as easily be made using chicken or vegetables. I've suggested my favorite vegetables for this recipe, but any vegetables you have on hand will work fine.

SAUCE

1½ cups Dairy Milk Alternative (page 173)

1½ tablespoons Gluten-Free Flour Mix (page 172)

1 large yellow onion, coarsely chopped

1 teaspoon minced fresh thyme, or ½ teaspoon dried

½ teaspoon minced fresh rosemary, or ¼ teaspoon dried

¼ teaspoon salt

3 cloves garlic, minced

½ cup red wine

2 tablespoons minced flat-leaf parsley

FILLING

2 tablespoons olive oil

1 pound lean ground lamb or beef

½ teaspoon salt

¼ teaspoon freshly ground black pepper

⅓ pound fresh mushrooms, quartered

2 large red bell peppers, seeded, ribbed, and coarsely chopped

¾ pound carrots, peeled and cut into 1-inch pieces (about 4 medium carrots)

½ cauliflower, broken into florets (about 1½ cups)

½ cup Chicken Stock (page 176)

Herbed Mashers (page 111), about 3 cups

TO PREPARE THE SAUCE: Combine the milk and flour in a blender, cover, and whirl at top speed, about 30 seconds. Heat a large saucepan over medium-high heat and add the onion, thyme, rosemary, salt, and 2 tablespoons of water. Steam-sauté, stirring frequently, until the onion is lightly browned, about 6 minutes. Stir in the garlic and wine and reduce the liquid by half, about 5 minutes. Gradually whisk in the milk mixture until a smooth sauce develops, about 3 minutes. (The sauce will be thick; do not allow it to boil.) Whisk in the parsley and season to taste.

TO PREPARE THE FILLING: Preheat the oven to 375°F. Heat the oil in a large skillet over medium-high heat. Season the lamb with the salt and pepper and add to the hot skillet, cooking until it is lightly browned, about 4 minutes. Add the vegetables and stock, and cook 4 to 5 minutes longer. Slowly add the sauce, stirring until fully incorporated. Transfer the mixture to a 4- to 5-quart casserole dish.

Spoon the mashed potatoes evenly over the lamb and vegetable mixture and bake until the sauce is bubbly, 40 to 45 minutes. Remove from the oven and let stand at room temperature for 10 minutes before serving.

sweet basil turkey loaf *with* mushroom sauce

Free of SOY NUT SUGAR OIL

SERVES 4

Nothing quite says comfort food like meat loaf smothered in creamy sauce, served with mashed potatoes. This turkey loaf makes a great casual weeknight dinner as well as terrific sandwiches the following day. It's a snap to prepare and can easily be assembled the night before. Extra-lean ground beef, ground lamb, or a combination of the two work equally well; just be sure to drain off the excess fat once the loaf is pulled from the oven.

1¼ **pounds ground turkey**

½ **pound carrots, peeled and minced, or grated**

1 **large yellow onion, minced**

2 **cloves garlic, minced**

1 **red bell pepper, seeded, ribbed, and minced**

¾ **cup stemmed and coarsely chopped fresh basil**

1 **cup gluten-free quick oats or quinoa flakes**

1 **large egg**

¼ **cup cream sherry**

¼ **teaspoon salt**

¼ **teaspoon freshly ground black pepper**

Mushroom Sauce (page 124)

TO PREPARE AND BAKE THE TURKEY LOAF: Preheat the oven to 350°F. Combine the turkey, carrots, onion, garlic, bell pepper, basil, oats, egg, sherry, salt, and pepper in a large bowl. With well-washed hands, mix the ingredients until well combined. Pat the mixture into an 8½ by 4½ by 2½-inch loaf pan and bake until lightly browned and the juices run clear, about 1½ hours.

TO SERVE THE LOAF: Allow the loaf to rest in the pan about 15 minutes before slicing. Slice the loaf into ¾-inch-thick slices and ladle the mushroom sauce on top. Serve immediately.

lamb tagine *with* dates

Free of EGG SOY NUT

SERVES 6

In Morocco, the term tagine *refers to slowly simmered meat, fish, and vegetable dishes that are highly aromatic and have both a sweet and savory flavor. These stews are prepared and served in an earthenware dish with a fitted lid.*

1 tablespoon canola oil

3 pounds boneless lamb shoulder or stew meat, cut into 1½-inch pieces

1 large yellow onion, coarsely chopped

⅓ cup chopped flat-leaf parsley

¼ cup chopped fresh cilantro

1 teaspoon ground cinnamon

1 teaspoon ground ginger

⅛ teaspoon crushed saffron threads

2 cups Vegetable Stock (page 177)

8 ounces pitted dates, quartered

2 tablespoons honey

1 (15-ounce) can chickpeas, rinsed and drained

2 oranges, peeled and cut into sections

¼ cup sliced almonds, toasted (see page 186)

½ teaspoon salt

½ teaspoon freshly ground black pepper

1½ cups cooked millet (page 181)

Heat the oil in a heavy Dutch oven over medium-high heat. Season the lamb with salt and pepper. In batches, add the lamb to the pot, searing until just brown, about 4 minutes per batch. Using a slotted spoon, transfer each batch of lamb to a bowl. Add the onion to the pot and sauté until tender, about 4 minutes. Mix in the parsley, cilantro, cinnamon, ginger, saffron, and vegetable stock. Return all of the lamb with its juices to the pot and bring to a rolling simmer. Cover and reduce the heat to low, and simmer until the lamb is tender, about 1½ hours. Add the dates, honey, and chickpeas to the lamb mixture, stirring to incorporate. Simmer until heated through, about 15 minutes. Transfer to a deep platter and garnish with orange sections and almonds. Serve atop the millet.

braised beef roast *over* herbed mashers *and* sautéed greens

SERVES 6

My husband Robert developed this simple recipe for braising beef.

The beef cuts that are best for braising are the tougher cuts, such as round, flank, and chuck. The chuck cuts are great for braising because of their wonderful flavor. They also have a generous amount of marbling that melts during the braising process, which allows for an internal basting that adds lots of moisture to the meat. Among the chuck cuts that make excellent brasiers are the chuck eye roast and the top blade chuck roast.

2 pounds beef pot roast (also called boneless chuck roast or cross-rib roast), about 3 inches thick

$^1/_2$ teaspoon salt

$^1/_2$ teaspoon freshly ground black pepper

1 tablespoon canola oil

1 medium yellow onion, finely chopped

2 cup carrots, finely chopped (about 3 carrots)

2 cups celery, finely chopped (about 5 stalks)

6 cloves garlic, minced

3 cups Chicken Stock (page 176)

2 bay leaves

$^1/_4$ cup chopped flat-leaf parsley, for garnish (optional)

Herbed Mashers (page 111), about 3 cups

Braised Greens with Caramelized Onion (page 114)

Trim any visible fat from the roast and sprinkle with salt and pepper. Heat the oil in a heavy Dutch oven over medium-high heat. Add the roast to the pan and brown the beef on all sides, 3 minutes per side, for a total of 12 minutes. Transfer the beef to a plate and set aside. Add the onions, carrots, and celery to the pan and sauté until the vegetables are softened, about 5 minutes. Add the garlic and $^1/_2$ cup of stock to deglaze the pan, scraping up the browned bits from the bottom of the pan. Add the remaining stock to the pan and stir to combine. Return the roast with its juices to the pan, bring to a boil, cover, and decrease the heat to low. Simmer for 3 hours. Transfer the roast to a cutting board to rest. Bring the braising mixture to a boil and reduce the liquid by one-third.

Slice the roast across the grain. Place a scoop of the mashed potatoes in the center of a bowl or plate, top with three slices of the beef, spoon the vegetables and braising liquid over the beef, and garnish with parsley. Serve with braised greens.

beef stroganoff

Free of EGG NUT SUGAR

SERVES 4

You'll be hard pressed to notice a difference between this stroganoff and traditional stroganoff made with sour cream. For a lighter version of this classic dish, try preparing it using lean turkey breast in place of the beef. If you have trouble finding gluten-free wide noodles, lasagna noodles cut 3/4 inch wide or fettucini noodles would work well in this recipe.

2 tablespoons olive oil

1 large yellow onion, coarsely chopped

1 pound boneless lean beef, sliced into 1-inch strips

$^1/_2$ teaspoon salt

$^1/_4$ teaspoon freshly ground black pepper

$^1/_3$ cup dry white wine

$^3/_4$ pound fresh white mushrooms, thinly sliced

1 teaspoon fresh thyme, or $^1/_2$ teaspoon dried

$^1/_4$ cup chopped flat-leaf parsley

$^1/_8$ teaspoon ground nutmeg

Lean Sour Cream (page 125)

1 (10-ounce) package wide gluten-free pasta

TO PREPARE THE STROGANOFF: Heat the olive oil in a large skillet over medium-high heat and sauté the onion until golden brown, about 5 minutes. Add the beef and season with salt and pepper. Sauté until evenly browned, 3 to 4 minutes. Add the wine, mushrooms, thyme, 2 tablespoons of the parsley, and nutmeg. Decrease the heat to medium-low, cover, and simmer for about 10 minutes, stirring occasionally. Add the sour cream and stir to blend. Simmer the stroganoff, uncovered, for about 5 minutes, stirring the mixture often and taking care not to boil the sauce.

Cook the pasta according to the package directions. Drain, rinse under warm running water, and drain again.

TO SERVE: Divide the pasta evenly among 4 individual plates and spoon the stroganoff mixture on top. Garnish with the remaining 2 tablespoons of chopped parsley.

vegetarian and companion dishes

Not just side dishes anymore, these versatile recipes make reducing the amount of animal proteins in our diets deliciously simple.

mushroom kale lasagna

Free of EGG SUGAR OIL

SERVES 6

The unexpected blend of mushrooms, kale, and creamy nut sauce make this distinctive lasagna so satisfying you won't miss the cheese.

2 cups Dairy Milk Alternative (page 173)

1 cup pine nuts or chopped cashews or a combination

1 tablespoon Gluten-Free Flour Mix (page 172) or arrowroot powder

1/4 cup water

1 large onion, finely chopped

4 cloves garlic, minced

1 teaspoon minced fresh thyme, or 1/4 teaspoon dried

1 teaspoon minced fresh oregano, or 1/4 teaspoon dried

1/4 teaspoon freshly ground black pepper

1 pound fresh white mushrooms, thinly sliced

1 bunch kale, stemmed and finely chopped

1 (12-ounce) package firm tofu, drained

3 cups Herbed Tomato Sauce (page 178), or 1 (28-ounce) jar of tomato sauce

1/4 cup minced flat-leaf parsley

1 (10-ounce) package gluten-free lasagna noodles (uncooked)

2 large tomatoes, thinly sliced

Chopped fresh parsley, for garnish (optional)

TO PREPARE THE NUT CREAM SAUCE: Combine the milk and nuts in a blender, then allow the nuts to soak for about 15 minutes. Add the flour, cover, and puree the mixture until smooth, about 1 minute.

TO PREPARE THE FILLING: Heat a large skillet over medium-high heat, add the onion and 2 tablespoons of water, and steam-sauté, stirring frequently, until the onion is tender, about 3 minutes. Add the garlic, thyme, oregano, and pepper, and sauté 1 minute longer. Add the mushrooms and remaining water and cook, stirring frequently, until the mushrooms are reduced by half in volume, about 6 minutes. Add the kale in batches until just wilted. Stir in the tomato sauce and parsley. Crumble the tofu and fold to blend with a spatula.

TO ASSEMBLE THE DISH: Preheat the oven to 400°F. Lightly coat a 9 by 13 by 2-inch baking dish with cooking spray. Ladle about 1/4 cup of the filling into the baking dish, spreading it evenly. Cover with a layer of noodles. Spread one quarter of the filling mixture on top of the pasta, distributing it evenly. Ladle 3/4 cup of cream sauce over the filling and top with another layer of noodles, filling, and sauce. Repeat for 2 more layers. Finish with sliced tomatoes. Cover tightly with aluminum foil, bake for 45 minutes, uncover, and bake for 20 minutes longer. Remove from the oven and let stand 15 minutes before slicing.

white bean fettuccini

Free of EGG SOY NUT SUGAR OIL

SERVES 4

Any white bean will work in this recipe but I am partial to cannellini beans. If broccolini is hard to find, you can substitute broccoli rabe (rapini), or stemmed, chopped kale or spinach. This vegetarian one-dish meal offers a hearty helping of fiber, vitamins, minerals, and protein.

1 large yellow onion, chopped

1$\frac{1}{2}$ cups sliced white mushrooms

1 red bell pepper, seeded, ribbed, and chopped

2 tablespoons Vegetable Stock (page 177)

1 teaspoon salt

4 cloves garlic, minced

2 teaspoons dried oregano

1 teaspoon dried thyme

$\frac{1}{8}$ teaspoon red chile flakes (optional)

2 cups Chopped Tomatoes (page 179)

$\frac{1}{2}$ cup white wine

2 cups cooked cannellini beans (see page 180)

2 bunches broccolini, cut into 1$\frac{1}{2}$-inch pieces

$\frac{1}{4}$ cup chopped flat-leaf parsley

1 (14-ounce) package gluten-free fettuccini noodles

TO COOK THE PASTA: Bring 3 quarts of water to a boil in a large saucepan over high heat. Cook about $\frac{3}{4}$ of a package of the fettuccini noodles, uncovered, according to the package directions, taking care not to overcook it.

TO PREPARE THE SAUCE: Meanwhile, in a large saucepan over medium-high heat, add the onion, mushrooms, bell pepper, stock, and salt, and cover and cook, stirring occasionally, until the mushrooms are softened, about 6 minutes. Add the garlic, oregano, thyme, and chile flakes, stirring to blend, about 1 minute. Add the chopped tomatoes and wine. Bring to a boil, cover, decrease the heat to low, and simmer for 15 minutes, stirring occasionally. Add the beans and broccolini and cook until just tender, 3 to 5 minutes. Add the parsley and stir to blend. Toss the sauce with the pasta and serve.

rustic heirloom pesto pizza

Free of EGG SOY SUGAR

MAKES ONE 12-INCH PIZZA

Bursting with fresh flavors this pizza was inspired by my summertime garden. Prepared simply with pesto and freshly sliced heirloom tomatoes warm from the vine, this pizza is one of my all time favorites.

Both this recipe and the Rustic Mushroom Pizza (page 98) use a gluten-free pizza crust that requires partial pre-baking, so it's important to have your sauce and topping ready to go. After you have tried these versions, experiment with your own favorite toppings.

SAUCE

1 cup Basil Pesto (page 129)

TOPPINGS

2 heirloom tomatoes (assorted red, yellow, purple, or green), sliced $1/2$ inch thick

Crispy Pizza Crust (page 140), or Traditional Pizza Crust (page 141)

Olive oil, for brushing (optional)

1 cup Creamy Macadamia Pine Nut Cheese (page 175)

$1/4$ teaspoon sea salt

$1/4$ teaspoon freshly ground black pepper

TO ASSEMBLE AND BAKE THE PIZZA: Preheat the oven to 425°F. Prepare and pre-bake the crust according to the recipe directions. Spoon the pesto sauce evenly onto the pre-baked crust leaving a $1/2$-inch border around the edge (brush the edge with olive oil, if using), and arrange the tomato slices over the top. Bake the pizza for 20 minutes, spoon several small dollops of the cheese onto the pizza, and continue baking until the crust is crisp and golden and the cheese is just warm, about 5 minutes longer. Remove from the oven and let stand for 5 minutes. Sprinkle with salt and pepper, slice, and serve.

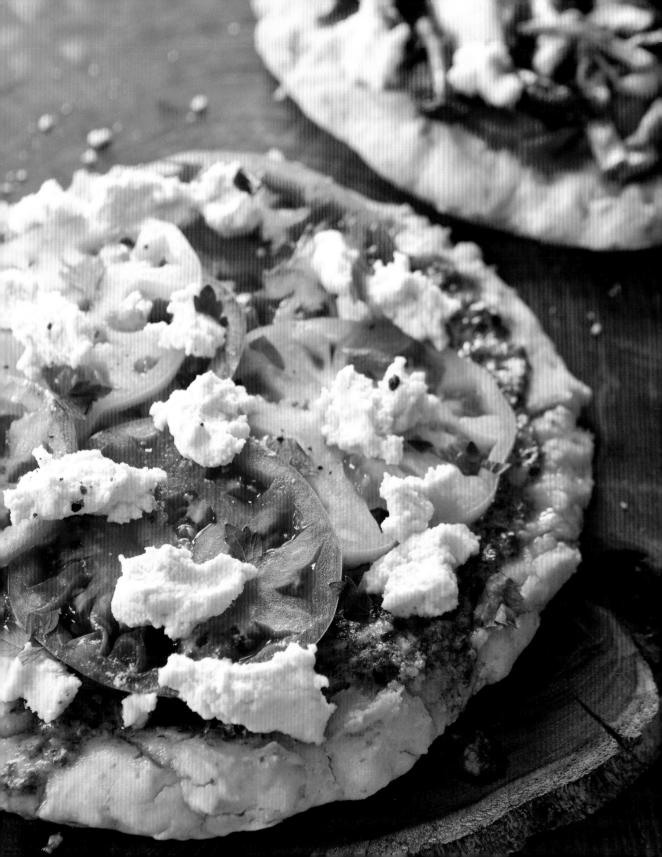

rustic mushroom pizza

MAKES ONE 12-INCH PIZZA

In Provence, France, they make a pizza crust with-out yeast, more like a tart shell, and top it with niçoise olives and anchovies. In Naples, Italy, they make a yeast pizza crust that is thin, light, and crisp. Often it's simply topped with a delicate but flavorful tomato sauce and seasonal toppings. Both pizza styles are unique and quite delicious.

SAUCE

2 cups Chopped Tomatoes (page 179), or 1 (14.5-ounce) can chopped tomatoes

3 cloves garlic, minced

TOPPINGS

1 medium yellow onion, thinly sliced

2 cups sliced assorted oyster mushrooms

1 teaspoon chopped fresh rosemary or thyme

$1/4$ teaspoon sea salt

$1/4$ teaspoon freshly ground black pepper

Additional suggested toppings: Lightly sautéed vegetables, such as spinach, thinly sliced potatoes, asparagus, and zucchini; chopped artichoke hearts, roasted red peppers, grilled eggplant, pitted green or black olives, capers, and fresh herbs

Crispy Pizza Crust (page 140) or Traditional Pizza Crust* (page 141)

Olive oil*, for brushing (optional)

1 cup Creamy Macadamia Pine Nut Cheese (page 175)

TO PREPARE THE SAUCE: Combine the chopped tomatoes and garlic in a saucepan over medium-high heat and bring to a boil. Decrease the heat to medium-low and simmer the tomatoes, uncovered, until they are reduced to $3/4$ cup, about 20 minutes. Remove from the heat and set aside to cool slightly.

TO PREPARE THE TOPPING: In a large skillet over medium-high heat, add the onion, mushrooms, rosemary, salt, and pepper and sauté until soft-ened and the liquid has evaporated, about 6 minutes; transfer to a plate.

TO ASSEMBLE AND BAKE THE PIZZA: Preheat the oven to 425°F. Prepare and bake the crust according to the recipe directions. Spoon the sauce evenly onto the pre-baked crust leaving a $1/2$-inch bor-der around the edge (brush the edge with olive oil, if using), and arrange the topping randomly but evenly over the top. Bake the pizza for 20 minutes, spoon several small dollops of the cheese onto the pizza, and continue baking until the crust is crisp and golden and the cheese is just warm, about 5 minutes longer. Remove from the oven and let stand for 5 minutes. Slice and serve.

creamy polenta

Free of EGG NUT SUGAR OIL

SERVES 4 TO 6

Jazz up any meal by spooning this rich-tasting polenta in the center of a plate and topping it with vegetables, tempeh, tofu, grilled poultry, meat, or fish. It's a snap to prepare and a healthy way to satisfy a craving for something rich and creamy.

6 ounces silken soft tofu, drained

2$^1/_4$ cups Dairy Milk Alternative (page 173)

3 tablespoons Date Syrup (page 189) or honey

$^1/_4$ teaspoon salt

$^1/_8$ teaspoon freshly ground black pepper

1 cup Vegetable Stock (page 177) or Chicken Stock (page 176)

1 cup medium ground yellow cornmeal

Chopped parsley, for garnish (optional)

In a large bowl, beat the tofu, $^1/_4$ cup of the milk, date syrup, salt, and pepper with an electric mixer until smooth and creamy, about 2 minutes. Set aside.

TO PREPARE THE POLENTA: In a large saucepan over medium-low heat, add the vegetable stock and remaining 2 cups of milk and bring to a simmer; do not boil. Decrease the heat to low and gradually add the cornmeal in a slow and steady stream, whisking constantly so that lumps do not form. Whisk the tofu mixture into the cornmeal and continue cooking until the polenta has thickened slightly, 15 to 20 minutes. Garnish with parsley. Serve hot.

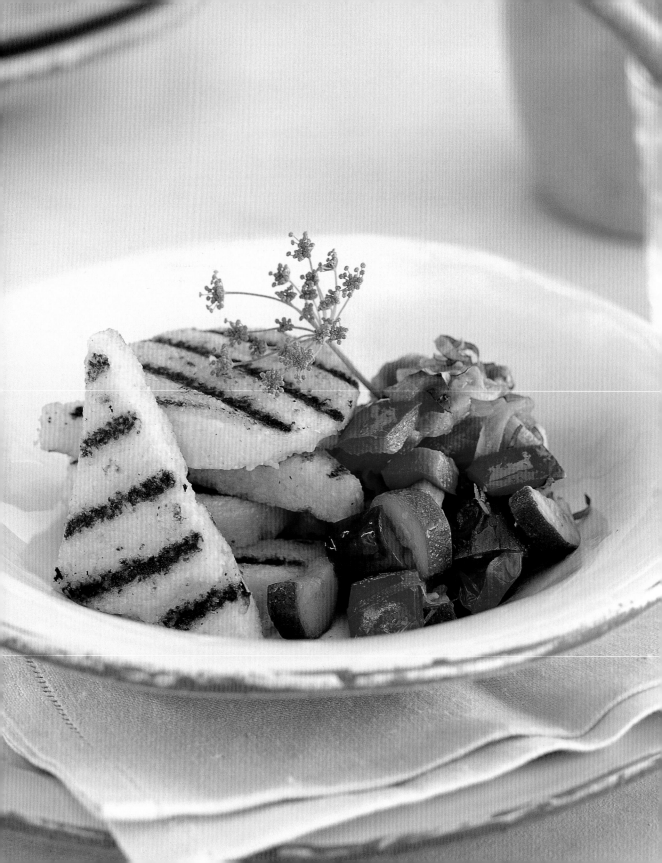

grilled polenta *with* vegetable ragout

Free of EGG SOY NUT SUGAR OIL*

YIELDS 16 SLICES

This colorful and flavorful dish is wonderful served alongside grilled chicken or fish. Accompanied by a salad, it makes a perfect light entrée.

POLENTA

6 cups Dairy Milk Alternative (page 173)

1¹/₂ teaspoons dried thyme

1 teaspoon salt

2 cups medium or coarse ground yellow cornmeal

Olive oil*, for brushing (optional)

RAGOUT

1¹/₄ cup Vegetable Stock (page 177)

1 large yellow onion, halved and thinly sliced

2 Japanese eggplants, or 1 small globe eggplant, cut into 1¹/₂-inch cubes

3 cloves garlic, minced

2 teaspoons salt

1 red bell pepper, seeded, ribbed, and chopped into ¹/₂-inch pieces

2 zucchinis, halved lengthwise and sliced ¹/₄ inch thick

2 cups Chopped Tomatoes (page 179), or 1 (14.5-ounce) can chopped tomatoes

¹/₃ cup hand-torn fresh basil leaves

¹/₂ teaspoon freshly ground black pepper

Basil sprigs, for garnish (optional)

TO PREPARE THE POLENTA: Combine the milk, thyme, and salt in a large saucepan over medium-high heat and bring to a simmer; do not boil. Decrease the heat to low and gradually add the cornmeal in a slow, steady stream, whisking constantly to avoid lumps. Continue whisking until the mixture thickens and pulls away from the side of the pan, about 20 minutes. Pour into a nonstick 8-inch loaf pan. Smooth the top with a spatula, gently pressing to compact the polenta. Allow to cool about 45 minutes. Cover with plastic wrap and refrigerate for 1 hour or overnight.

TO PREPARE THE RAGOUT: Heat a large skillet over medium-high heat, add the onion and 1 table-spoon of the stock, and steam-sauté for 3 minutes. Add the remaining stock, eggplant, garlic, and salt, and sauté, stirring often, about 5 minutes. Add the bell pepper, zucchini, tomatoes, basil, and pepper, and sauté for 3 minutes. Cover and simmer the vegetables over low heat, stirring occasionally, until the vegetables are just soft-ened, about 5 minutes. Remove from the heat and set aside. Season to taste.

Preheat the grill or broiler. Turn the polenta out onto a cutting board and slice into sixteen ¹/₂-inch-thick pieces. Then, slice each piece diag-onally, forming 2 triangles. Transfer to a cookie sheet and brush both sides lightly with olive oil.

continued

Grill or broil each side until lightly browned, 1 to 3 minutes. Transfer to serving plates. To serve as a starter or side dish, arrange 2 slices of the grilled polenta on a plate and spoon the ragout on top, garnishing with basil sprigs. As an entrée, arrange 4 slices per plate.

corn soufflé

Free of SOY NUT OIL

SERVES 4 TO 6

Delicate and flavorful, this soufflé is easy to prepare and makes an elegant addition to grilled chicken or vegetables. The key ingredient—a must for this recipe—is the vanilla-flavored dairy milk alternative.

---

3 cups vanilla Dairy Milk Alternative (page 173)

1 teaspoon salt

1 cup finely ground yellow cornmeal

2 tablespoons sugar

3/4 cup white corn kernels, fresh (about 2 ears) or frozen

6 large eggs, separated

1/4 teaspoon cream of tartar

Preheat the oven to 375°F. Lightly grease a 2-quart soufflé dish with the canola oil. Combine the milk and salt in a large saucepan over medium-high heat and bring to a simmer, taking care not to boil the liquid. Decrease the heat to low. Gradually add the cornmeal in a slow and steady stream, whisking constantly so that lumps do not form, until the mixture begins to thicken, 2 to 3 minutes. Add the sugar, whisking until the sugar dissolves and the mixture is smooth, about 1 minute. Stir in the corn. Remove the mixture from the heat and allow to cool slightly, stirring occasionally, about 10 minutes.

Meanwhile, in a large bowl, whisk the egg yolks until well blended. Gradually add the cornmeal mixture to the yolks and stir to blend.

Using an electric mixer on high speed, beat the egg whites and cream of tartar in a medium bowl until they form soft peaks. With a rubber spatula, gently fold the whites into the cornmeal mixture until just combined. Do not overmix or the soufflé will not rise. Pour the mixture into the prepared soufflé dish and bake until the soufflé rises and turns golden brown, 35 to 40 minutes. Serve immediately.

cheesy mac 'n' nut cheese

Free of EGG* SUGAR OIL

SERVES 6

For the kid in all of us—this delicious version of mac 'n' cheese does not rely on store-bought cheese for its ooey-gooey richness. Instead, the cashews provide a rich buttery taste balanced by the cheesy flavor from the nutritional yeast flakes. Enjoy this recipe with or without the breadcrumb topping; either way, it is very satisfying.

1 (16-ounce) package of gluten-free elbow macaroni

$^1/_2$ cup raw cashew pieces

2 cups Dairy Milk Alternative (page 173)

1 red bell pepper, seeded, ribbed, and coarsely chopped

1 tablespoon arrowroot powder

1 teaspoon freshly squeezed lemon juice

1 teaspoon dry mustard powder

1 teaspoon turmeric

1 teaspoon salt

$^1/_2$ teaspoon onion powder

$^1/_8$ teaspoon white pepper

$^1/_4$ teaspoon garlic powder

1 cup nutritional yeast flakes

$^3/_4$ cup Gluten-Free Bread Cumbs* (page 185), 2 to 3 slices (optional)

Cook the macaroni according to package directions; do not overcook. Meanwhile, prepare the sauce.

TO PREPARE THE SAUCE: Place the cashews in a bowl of warm water to cover, and soak for 30 minutes or up to 4 hours. Drain, rinse, and drain again. Add the milk, cashews, bell pepper, arrowroot, lemon juice, mustard, turmeric, salt, onion, white pepper, garlic, and nutritional yeast to a blender. Cover and puree until smooth, about 1 minute.

TO ASSEMBLE THE DISH: Transfer the pureed mixture to a large saucepan. Whisking constantly, bring the mixture to a simmer over medium heat until a smooth sauce develops and thickens, about 4 minutes. Add the drained macaroni to the sauce, stirring with a spoon until incorporated and heated though. Serve immediately; or for breadcrumb version, preheat the broiler. Position the oven rack 6 inches from the heat source. Transfer the macaroni to an 8 by 8 by 2-inch glass baking dish and evenly distribute bread crumbs on top. Broil until the bread crumbs are lightly browned, about 3 minutes. Watch them carefully so they don't burn. Serve hot.

blackstrap beans

Free of EGG   SOY   NUT   OIL

SERVES 6

Team these calcium-rich beans with barbecued dishes, or use them as a topping for baked potatoes or Creamy Polenta (page 99). Blackstrap molasses is a good source of iron, calcium, and potassium. Add a generous serving of sautéed greens and presto, you'll have a protein- and nutrient-packed meal!

2 large yellow onions, chopped

1 green bell pepper, seeded, ribbed, and coarsely chopped

3 cloves garlic, minced

1³/₄ cups Chopped Tomatoes (page 179), or 1 (14.5-ounce) can chopped tomatoes

³/₄ cup Vegetable Stock (page 177) or water

¹/₃ cup blackstrap molasses

2 tablespoons apple cider vinegar

1 tablespoon Worcestershire sauce

1 teaspoon dry mustard

¹/₂ teaspoon salt

¹/₄ teaspoon freshly ground black pepper

3 cups cooked great Northern beans, cannellini beans, or kidney beans (see page 180), or 1¹/₂ (15-ounce) cans, drained and rinsed

TO PREPARE THE BEANS: Set a large, heavy pot over medium-high heat. Add the onion, bell pepper, garlic, and ¹/₄ cup of the vegetable stock to the pot and sauté until tender, stirring often, about 8 minutes. Stir in the tomatoes, remaining stock, molasses, vinegar, Worcestershire sauce, mustard, salt, and pepper until the sugar has dissolved. Add the beans, stirring to combine. Decrease the heat to medium-low and simmer, uncovered, stirring occasionally, until the mixture begins to thicken, about 20 minutes. Taste to correct the seasonings.

richly spiced dal

SERVES 6

Lentil cooking times vary depending on the type of lentil used. This recipe calls for lentils that have been hulled, thus reducing their cooking time. If using other varieties such as common brown, Grande, Le Puy, Eston, Pardina, or Beluga, increase the cooking time by another 15 minutes. Serve with brown, red, or black rice and a side of greens.

1 tablespoon coconut oil or olive oil

1 yellow onion, finely chopped

1 teaspoon cumin seeds

$1/4$ teaspoon ground cardamom

4 cloves garlic, minced

4 cups Vegetable Stock (page 177)

2 cups red lentils (Red Chief, Crimson, Canary/Sutter's Gold)

$1^1/2$ cups Chopped Tomatoes with their juice, or 1 (14.5-ounce) can chopped tomatoes

2 tablespoons minced fresh ginger

1 teaspoon ground turmeric

1 teaspoon salt

$1/3$ cup chopped fresh cilantro

TO PREPARE THE LENTILS: Place the lentils on a clean, flat surface, preferably light in color to aid in sorting. Sort through the lentils and discard any pebbles or chaff. Place the sorted lentils in a fine-mesh strainer and rinse with cold running water; drain.

TO PREPARE THE DAL: Heat the oil in a large, heavy 5-quart pan over medium-high heat and sauté the onion until golden brown, about 5 minutes. Add the cumin, cardamom, and garlic to the pan and stir until the spices are just fragrant, about 2 minutes. Add the stock, tomatoes, lentils, ginger, turmeric, and salt. Bring to a boil over high heat; reduce the heat to low, cover, and simmer, stirring often, until lentils are soft, about 15 minutes. Toss with the cilantro and serve over rice.

pan-seared tofu

SERVES 4

Once you've marinated the tofu, you can use the remaining marinade to make a savory sauce by reducing it in a saucepan, and top it with Apple Mango Chutney (page 134).

2 (12-ounce) packages firm or extra-firm tofu, drained

¹⁄₄ cup gluten-free tamari

¹⁄₄ cup freshly squeezed orange juice

2 tablespoons dry white wine or sake

2 tablespoons minced green onion, white and green parts

2 teaspoons dark sesame oil

3 cloves garlic, minced

1 teaspoon freshly squeezed lemon juice

2 teaspoons peeled, minced fresh ginger, or 1 teaspoon ground

1 teaspoon freshly ground black pepper

1 tablespoon coconut oil

Apple Mango Chutney (page 134), for serving

TO PREPARE THE TOFU: Place the tofu atop several layers of paper towels on a large plate. Cover the tofu with additional paper towels and then another plate. Place something heavy on top of the plate to weigh it, such as 3 or 4 cans of soup. Allow the tofu to drain about 30 minutes. Replace the wet towels with dry ones and continue to press the tofu for 30 minutes longer. Cut the tofu into 1-inch-thick slabs.

TO MARINATE THE TOFU: Whisk the tamari, orange juice, wine, green onion, sesame oil, garlic, lemon juice, ginger, and pepper in a bowl until blended. Place the drained tofu slabs side by side in a shallow container with a tight-fitting lid. Pour the marinade over the tofu, making sure the tofu is immersed in the marinade. Cover and refrigerate at least 24 hours and up to 48 hours.

TO SEAR THE TOFU: Heat the coconut oil in a sauté pan over medium-high heat until very hot. Lift the tofu out of the marinade, reserving the marinade, and place in the hot skillet, partially covering the skillet with a lid to lessen spattering. Sear the tofu until dark brown, about 3 minutes. Turn over with a spatula and cook the other side until dark brown, 2 to 3 minutes longer. Transfer to a plate.

TO MAKE THE SAUCE: Pour the marinade into the hot skillet. Bring the marinade to a boil, whisking constantly. Decrease the heat to medium-low, and reduce the marinade by one-third. Serve the tofu with a small amount of sauce spooned on top.

the **dairy-free** and **gluten-free** kitchen

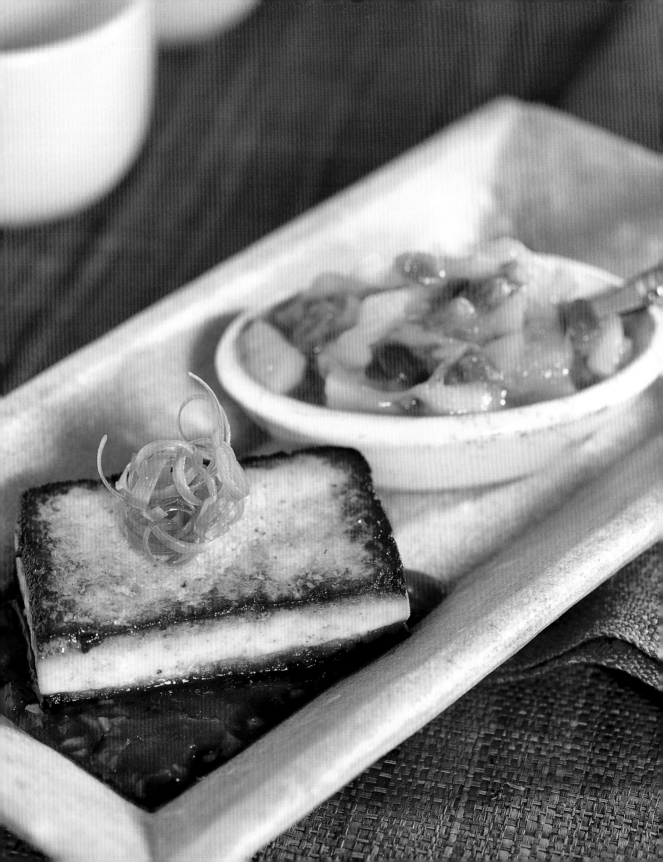

portobello risotto

Free of EGG SOY NUT SUGAR

SERVES 4

The rich, full-bodied flavor of portobello mushrooms and the creamy texture of the rice makes this dish deeply satisfying. Portobellos are fully grown crimini mushrooms with a natural meatiness that acts as a nice substitute for animal proteins. For a simple variation, try tossing in 1/3 cup of lightly toasted pine nuts, sunflower seeds, or almonds before serving. If added any sooner, the nuts will absorb moisture and lose their crunch.

3 tablespoons olive oil

3 large portobello mushrooms

3 cloves garlic, minced

1/2 teaspoon salt

1/4 teaspoon freshly ground black pepper

1 yellow onion, finely chopped

2 cups Arborio or carnaroli rice

6 sprigs thyme, or 1/2 teaspoon dried

1/2 cup dry white wine

6 cups Vegetable Stock (page 177) or Chicken Stock (page 176)

1 tablespoon freshly squeezed lemon juice (about 1 lemon)

TO PREPARE THE MUSHROOMS: With the gills facing up, place the mushrooms on a cutting board and gently twist to remove the stems. Using a spoon, lightly scrape out the black gills and discard. Slice the mushrooms in half and thinly slice the caps into 1 1/2-inch-thick slices. Heat 2 tablespoons of the olive oil in a large skillet over medium-high heat and sauté the mushrooms, garlic, salt, and pepper, until the mushrooms are softened, about 3 minutes; set aside.

TO MAKE THE RISOTTO: In a large saucepan over medium heat, add the remaining 1 tablespoon of the oil and sauté the onion until soft and golden, about 8 minutes. Add the rice and thyme to the onion and, using a wooden spoon, toss to coat.

Add the wine and stir until the liquid has been absorbed. Add the stock to the rice mixture, a ladleful at a time, stirring constantly after each addition until the liquid is absorbed. Continue adding the stock, a ladleful at a time, until a creamy sauce develops and all of the remaining stock has been used; this should take 20 to 25 minutes. Add the mushroom mixture with its juices to the rice and stir to incorporate. Taste and correct the seasonings. Serve immediately.

scalloped potatoes

SERVES 4 TO 6

Elegant and satisfying, these potatoes make a scrumptious addition to any meat or fish entrée. I particularly enjoy pairing them with the Peppered Pork Tenderloin in Mustard Cream Sauce (page 87) or the Halibut in Swiss Chard Wraps (page 72). Onions are slowly sautéed with bay to draw out the subtle flavor, then layered with thin slices of potato. A touch of nutmeg sweetens the delicate cream sauce. This recipe is well suited to a mandoline which will cut the prep time in half.

1 tablespoon olive oil

2 medium yellow onions, thinly sliced

1 bay leaf

1/2 teaspoon dried thyme

3 cloves garlic, minced

1 tablespoon Gluten-Free Flour Mix (page 172)

2 pounds russet potatoes, peeled and thinly sliced

1 cup Dairy Milk Alternative (page 173)

1 cup plain dairy-free yogurt*

1 teaspoon salt

1/2 teaspoon ground nutmeg

1/4 teaspoon freshly ground black pepper

1/4 teaspoon paprika

Preheat oven to 425°F.

TO PREPARE THE ONIONS: Heat the olive oil in a large sauté pan over medium-low heat. Add the onion, bay leaf, and thyme and sauté until the onion is lightly caramelized, 10 to 12 minutes. Add the garlic and sauté for 1 minute longer. Remove from the heat, discard the bay leaf, sprinkle the onion with the flour, and stir to blend. Set aside.

TO ASSEMBLE THE DISH: Coat the inside of an 8 by 11 by 2-inch baking dish with olive oil. Arrange one-third of the potatoes in the prepared dish in a single layer, slightly overlapping the edges of the potatoes. Spread one-half of the onion mixture on top of the potatoes. Add another layer, using one-third of the potatoes and the remaining onions. For the final layer, evenly distribute the remaining potatoes.

In a large bowl, whisk together the milk, yogurt, salt, nutmeg, and pepper to blend. Pour this mixture over the potatoes to coat them completely. Using the back of a fork, lightly press down on the potatoes to compact the layers. Finish by sprinkling with the paprika. Bake, uncovered, for 30 minutes. Decrease the oven temperature to 350°F and continue baking until the top is golden brown and the potatoes are tender, 35 to 40 minutes longer. Remove from the oven and let stand 15 minutes before serving.

yam *and* potato mashers

SERVES 6

Any yam will work well in this recipe though my preference is garnet yams. Do not use white sweet potatoes, as they do not mash well and instead tend to turn gluey.

2¹/₂ pounds garnet yams, peeled and cut into 2-inch pieces

1 pound Yukon Gold, Yellow Finn, or russet potatoes, peeled and cut into 2-inch pieces

¹/₂ teaspoon salt

2 tablespoons olive oil* (optional)

¹/₈ teaspoon freshly ground black pepper

Place the potatoes and yams in a large pot with enough water to cover by 2 inches; add ¹/₄ teaspoon of the salt. Bring to a boil and cook until the potatoes break apart easily with a fork, 25 to 30 minutes. Place a colander over a bowl and drain, reserving the cooking liquid.

Transfer to a large bowl. Using a potato masher, smash the olive oil, 1 cup of the reserved cooking liquid, the remaining ¹/₄ teaspoon of the salt, and pepper, until the potatoes are fluffy. If needed, gradually add a little more of the cooking liquid, about ¹/₄ cup at a time, until the desired consistency is achieved. Season to taste. Serve hot.

herbed mashers

Free of EGG SOY NUT SUGAR OIL*

SERVES 6

If you use a milk alternative in place of the cooking liquid in this recipe, choose from almond, soy, or hemp milk. Rice milk reacts differently with heat and if you don't serve the potatoes immediately, it will thin, leaving the potatoes soupy.

1 teaspoon salt

1 cup stemmed, thinly sliced fresh basil leaves, tightly packed

$1/2$ cup stemmed, thinly sliced fresh spinach leaves, tightly packed

$1/4$ cup stemmed, chopped flat-leaf parsley

4 pounds Yukon Gold or Yellow Finn potatoes, quartered

2 tablespoons olive oil* (optional)

$1/8$ teaspoon freshly ground black pepper

$1/4$ cup minced fresh chives (about 2 bunches)

Place the potatoes in a large pot with enough water to cover by about 1 inch; add $1/4$ teaspoon of the salt. Bring the water to a boil. Place the basil, spinach, and parsley in a fine-mesh strainer and blanch the greens in the boiling water for about 1 minute. Remove the strainer and place it under cold running water to stop the cooking. Drain and set aside. Add the potatoes to the boiling water and cook until they break apart easily with a fork, 25 to 30 minutes. Place a colander over a bowl and drain the potatoes, catching and reserving the cooking liquid.

Using a potato masher, smash the potatoes until fluffy, adding the olive oil, the remaining add $3/4$ teaspoon of salt, pepper, and $13/4$ cups of the reserved cooking liquid, $1/2$ cup at a time. If needed, gradually add a little more of the cooking liquid, about $1/4$ cup at a time, until the desired consistency is achieved. Add the chives and blanched greens and stir until just incorporated. Season to taste. Serve hot.

wild lemon pilaf *with* currants

SERVES 6

With its buttery fragrance and subtle, almost nutty flavor, basmati rice pairs perfectly with the rich texture of wild rice. This pilaf recipe, infused with lemon and lightly sweetened with plump currants, is delicious alongside the Baked Salmon in Parchment (page 69).

3 cups water

$^2/_3$ cup wild rice, rinsed and drained

1 pound leeks, white and pale green parts only, julienned

$1^1/_3$ cups basmati or jasmine rice

$3^3/_4$ cups Vegetable Stock (page 177) or Chicken Stock (page 176)

$^1/_4$ cup freshly squeezed lemon juice (about 2 lemons)

1 tablespoon chopped lemon zest (2 to 3 lemons)

$^1/_3$ cup dried currants

$^1/_2$ teaspoon salt

$^1/_4$ teaspoon freshly ground black pepper

$^1/_4$ cup slivered almonds, toasted (see page 186)

TO PREPARE THE WILD RICE: Bring the water to a boil in a saucepan over medium-high heat. Add the wild rice. Decrease the heat to medium-low and simmer, uncovered, for about 15 minutes. Remove from the heat and drain in a fine-mesh strainer. Rinse under warm running water and drain again.

TO PREPARE THE PILAF: Heat a large saucepan over medium-high heat. Add the leeks and 2 tablespoons of stock; steam-sauté, stirring frequently, until the leeks are soft but not brown, about 3 minutes. Mix in the wild and basmati rice, tossing to combine. Stir in the vegetable stock, lemon juice, zest, currants, salt, and pepper. Bring the mixture to a boil, stirring occasionally. Cover, decrease the heat to low, and simmer until the liquid is absorbed and the rice is tender, about 35 minutes. Mix in the almonds and serve.

sautéed spinach *with* toasted pine nuts

Free of   SOY   SUGAR   OIL*

SERVES 4

Spinach, like many leafy greens, can be cooked with the water remaining on its leaves, eliminating the need for cooking oil. Simply wash and drain it briefly, then add it to a hot sauté pan and you'll have a nutritious vegetable in no time! To reduce the prep time, purchase pre-washed organic spinach, and remember, cooking reduces the volume of spinach significantly.

½ cup coarse Gluten-Free Bread Crumbs (page 185)

3 tablespoons pine nuts

1 clove garlic, thinly sliced

1 pound fresh spinach, stemmed and coarsely chopped

½ cup lightly packed fresh basil, thinly sliced

Zest of 1 lemon

⅛ teaspoon freshly ground black pepper

Olive oil* (optional)

Crushed red pepper flakes (optional)

In a large sauté pan over medium-high heat, combine the bread crumbs, pine nuts, and garlic; cook, stirring, until just fragrant, taking care not to burn the nuts. Transfer to a plate and set aside. To the sauté pan, add the rinsed spinach in batches and cook until just wilted, about 2 minutes. Transfer the spinach to a bowl and add the basil, lemon zest, pepper, and pine nut mixture; toss to incorporate, and serve immediately. If desired, top with a drizzle of olive oil and sprinkling of red pepper flakes.

braised greens
with caramelized onion

Free of EGG SOY NUT SUGAR OIL

SERVES 4

This is one of my favorite ways to cook greens. The sweetness from the caramelized onion and vinegar reduction marry beautifully with any type of mild, earthy, or leafy green. Choose from broccoli rabe, kale (curly leaf or lacinato), mustard greens, beet greens, bok choy, or Swiss chard; all will work equally well in this recipe.

---

1 large red onion, halved and thinly sliced

2 tablespoons Vegetable Stock (page 177), plus more if needed

2 tablespoons red wine vinegar or balsamic vinegar

¼ teaspoon salt

1 clove garlic, thinly sliced

1 pound lacinato kale (dinosaur kale), center stem removed and leaves thinly sliced

Heat a large saucepan over medium heat; add the onion, salt, and 1 tablespoon of the stock. Steam-saute, stirring frequently, until the onion is lightly browned and the liquid has evaporated, about 5 minutes. Reduce the heat to medium-low, add the garlic and the remaining 1 tablespoon of stock, and cook until the onion is soft, about 10 minutes. If the onion begins to stick to the pan, add more stock, 1 tablespoon at a time, to deglaze the pan.

Add the vinegar to the pan and increase the heat to medium-high. Add the kale plus ¼ cup of water and cook, stirring, until the kale begins to soften, about 3 minutes. As the liquid evaporates, add another ¼ cup of water and cook until the kale is tender, about 3 minutes longer. Serve immediately.

lemon-garlic crusted leeks

Free of SOY NUT SUGAR

SERVES 4 TO 6

This fabulous trio of leek, lemon, and garlic is a match made in heaven. Crunchy and flavorful, these leeks make a delicious accessory to the main course. Leeks often harbor a fair amount of grit between their delicate white layers, so be sure to rinse them thoroughly.

---

6 medium leeks, white and pale green parts only

1 large lemon

2 tablespoons olive oil

4 cloves garlic, minced

$^1/_3$ cup Gluten-Free Bread Crumbs (page 185)

$^1/_4$ teaspoon salt

$^1/_4$ teaspoon freshly ground black pepper

TO PREPARE THE LEEKS: Trim the leeks, discarding the dark green leaves. Cut the leeks in half lengthwise and rinse well in cold water, being careful to keep the halves intact. Set aside.

TO PREPARE THE LEMON AND STEAM THE LEEKS: Zest the lemon into a small bowl and set aside. Cut the zested lemon in half and squeeze 1 teaspoon of juice into the zest. Squeeze the remaining lemon juice into a large pot equipped with a steaming basket. Add the 2 lemon halves to the pot, along with enough water to steam the leeks. Place the pot over high heat and bring the water to a boil. Arrange the leeks, cut-sides up, in the basket. Fit the basket in the pot, cover, and steam the leeks until slightly tender, 10 to 15 minutes. Drain well. Arrange the leeks, cut-sides up, on a lightly oiled baking sheet and set aside. The leeks can be prepared 1 day ahead. If preparing them ahead, cover and refrigerate.

TO PREPARE THE TOPPING: In a saucepan over medium heat, sauté the garlic in the olive oil until tender, about 2 minutes. Remove the saucepan from the heat and add the bread crumbs, lemon zest, salt, and pepper. Stir until blended.

TO COOK THE LEEKS: Preheat the broiler. Position the oven rack 3 to 4 inches from the heat source. Using a teaspoon, spoon the breadcrumb mixture onto the cut side of the leeks and gently pat the mixture down with the back of the spoon. Broil until the leeks are golden brown, about 3 minutes. Watch them carefully so they do not burn. Serve hot or warm.

roasted brussels sprouts
in a balsamic reduction

Free of EGG SOY NUT SUGAR

SERVES 4

Brussels sprouts are a member of the cabbage family and share many of the same health-enhancing attributes, including an ample amount of antioxidants, vitamins, and minerals. This festive vegetable is simple to make and quick to assemble. By reducing the balsamic vinegar you concentrate the flavors creating a versatile, aromatic, and sweet sauce that is delicious drizzled over vegetables, fruit, or meats.

1¹/₂ **pounds brussels sprouts (about 4 cups)**

6 **cloves garlic, peeled**

2 **tablespoons olive oil**

¹/₂ **teaspoon coarse salt**

¹/₂ **teaspoon freshly ground black pepper**

1 **cup balsamic vinegar**

TO PREPARE THE BRUSSELS SPROUTS: Preheat the oven to 425°F. Trim off the stem ends and discard any yellow or discolored outer leaves. Cut the brussels sprouts in half lengthwise. Place them in a colander, rinse, and pat dry. Combine the brussels sprouts, garlic, olive oil, salt, and pepper in a large bowl, and toss thoroughly to coat.

Transfer the sprouts to a rimmed baking sheet, and spread them out in a single layer. Roast, shaking the pan occasionally to keep the vegetables from sticking, until just browned on the outside and tender on the inside, 15 to 20 minutes. Meanwhile, prepare the balsamic reduction.

TO PREPARE THE BALSAMIC REDUCTION: Place the balsamic vinegar in a small sauté pan with sloping sides over medium-high heat; whisking constantly, reduce the vinegar by one-half to three-quarters.

TO ASSEMBLE THE DISH: Transfer the roasted brussels sprouts to a bowl, drizzle with the balsamic reduction, and toss to coat. Serve warm.

roasted vegetable medley

SERVES 6

I enjoy serving these vegetables throughout the summer and early fall, when the squash is at its peak. You can use any combination of vegetables, but it's important to cut them to a uniform size so they cook at the same pace. This colorful medley can be served hot atop Yam and Potato Mashers (page 110) as a colorful vegan dish, with roasted meats, or as a cold salad.

2 carrots, peeled, halved lengthwise, and cut into 1-inch pieces

2 red bell peppers, seeded, ribbed, and cut into 1-inch pieces

2 zucchinis, ends trimmed, halved lengthwise, and cut into 1-inch pieces

2 yellow crookneck squash, ends trimmed, halved lengthwise, and cut into 1-inch pieces

$1/2$ pound red cabbage, cut into 1-inch cubes

$1/2$ pound cauliflower, cut into florets

2 medium yellow onions, cut into 1-inch pieces

2 tablespoons olive oil

1 tablespoon balsamic vinegar

1 tablespoon minced fresh rosemary, or 1 teaspoon dried

2 teaspoons minced fresh thyme, or $1/2$ teaspoon dried

2 cloves garlic, minced

$1/2$ teaspoon salt

$1/4$ teaspoon freshly ground black pepper

Preheat the oven to 350°F. Combine the carrots, bell pepper, squash, cabbage, cauliflower, and onion in a large bowl. Whisk the olive oil, vinegar, rosemary, thyme, garlic, salt, and pepper in a small bowl until blended. Pour the oil mixture over the vegetables and toss thoroughly to coat.

Transfer the vegetables to a shallow roasting pan and spread them out in a single layer. Roast the vegetables for 20 minutes, turn them with a spatula, and continue roasting until they are tender and brown but not soft, 20 to 30 minutes longer. Transfer the vegetables to a bowl to serve.

spicy roasted cauliflower

Free of   SOY   NUT   SUGAR   OIL*

SERVES 4

This is hands down my family's favorite way to eat cauliflower. Depending of your tastes this recipe can be made as spicy as you like by simply using hotter versions of the curry powder, paprika, or more red pepper flakes. For those who do not want to turn up the heat, use the mild versions of these spices and reduce or omit the red pepper flakes. Cauliflower is an excellent source of vitamin C, calcium, and potassium and is the most easily digestible member of the cabbage family.

1 large head of cauliflower, cut into florets

3 carrots, peeled, halved lengthwise, and cut into 1-inch pieces

1 medium russet potato, peeled and cut into 1-inch pieces

1 yellow onion, cut into 1-inch pieces

$1/2$ cup Gluten-Free Bread Crumbs (page 185)

2 tablespoons olive oil* (optional)

$1/2$ teaspoon ground turmeric

$1/2$ teaspoon paprika or smoked paprika

$1/2$ teaspoon yellow curry powder

$1/4$ teaspoon garlic powder

$1/4$ teaspoon salt

$1/8$ teaspoon crushed red pepper flakes, more or less to taste

Preheat the oven to 425°F. Oil a shallow 12 by 17-inch roasting pan with olive oil and set aside. Place the cauliflower, carrots, potato, onion and bread crumbs in a large bowl. Combine the turmeric, paprika, curry, garlic powder, salt, and pepper flakes in a small bowl and stir to blend. If using olive oil drizzle over the vegetables. Sprinkle the spice mixture over the vegetables and, using your hands, toss thoroughly to coat.

Transfer the vegetables to a shallow roasting pan and spread them out in a single layer. Roast the vegetables for 20 minutes, turn them with a spatula, reduce the heat to 350°F, and continue roasting until they are tender and just browned, about 15 minutes longer. Transfer the vegetables to a bowl to serve.

sauces, salsas, and spreads

When cooking dairy- and gluten-free, it's important to use flavor enhancers. Well-chosen sauces, salsas, and condiments make a simple dish sparkle. These sauces, salsas, and spreads are modest by themselves, but enhance and transform other foods.

pepper bean sauce

Free of EGG SOY NUT SUGAR

MAKES 4 CUPS

Spicy or mild, this bean sauce is a colorful addition to grilled fish or chicken. It can be made up to 1 day ahead and stored in a covered nonmetallic container in the refrigerator.

1 tablespoon olive oil

1 large yellow onion, chopped

3 cloves garlic, minced

2 cups Chicken Stock (page 176) or Vegetable Stock (page 177)

1 large red bell pepper, roasted, and cut into quarters (see page 182)

2 cups garbanzo beans, cooked and drained (see page 180)

$1/4$ cup dry white wine

$1^1/2$ tablespoons yellow curry powder

$1/8$ teaspoon crushed red pepper flakes

$1/4$ teaspoon salt

1 teaspoon seasoned rice vinegar

Heat the olive oil in a large sauté pan over medium-high heat and sauté the onion until tender, about 3 minutes. Add the garlic and sauté for about 1 minute. Stir in the chicken stock, roasted pepper, beans, wine, curry powder, red pepper flakes, and salt. Bring to a boil, decrease the heat to low, and simmer until the beans break apart easily with a fork, 25 to 30 minutes. Ladle the ingredients into a blender, cover tightly, and puree until smooth, about 2 minutes. Transfer the sauce back to the saucepan, stir in the rice vinegar, and warm over low heat, stirring occasionally, until the sauce is heated through. Taste and correct the seasonings. Serve warm.

black bean sauce

Free of EGG SOY NUT SUGAR OIL

MAKES 3 CUPS

This rich and robust sauce has a touch of lime juice, which adds a delicate, piquant flavor to the beans. To use the sauce as a delicious dip for tortilla chips, simply decrease the cooking liquid to $1/2$ cup when pureeing the mixture and don't bother to warm it up. Canned beans are not suitable for this recipe, because both the flavor and the color of the sauce would be compromised.

2 cups cooked black beans (see page 180)

1 cup reserved black bean cooking liquid

$1/2$ cup finely chopped yellow onion

3 cloves garlic, minced

1 jalapeño pepper, seeded and minced, more or less to taste

3 tablespoons freshly squeezed lime juice

$1/2$ teaspoon ground cumin

$1/2$ teaspoon salt

$1/8$ teaspoon freshly ground black pepper

Combine the beans, reserved liquid, onion, garlic, jalapeño, lime juice, cumin, salt, and pepper in a blender. Cover tightly and puree for 1 minute. The sauce will appear smooth with dark flecks throughout. Transfer the pureed mixture to a saucepan. Set the saucepan over medium-low heat and stir occasionally until the sauce is heated through, about 8 minutes. Take care not to boil the sauce. Taste and correct the seasonings. Serve warm or at room temperature.

sun-dried tomato cream

Free of EGG NUT SUGAR

MAKES 1½ CUPS

This brilliant sauce makes a zesty addition to grilled chicken or fish. Add a tablespoon to grain dishes, such as the Creamy Polenta (page 99), or spoon it over poached eggs on toast for a bright and flavorful finish.

1 cup dry white wine

¼ cup white wine vinegar

1½ tablespoons freshly squeezed lemon juice (about 1 lemon)

8 whole black peppercorns

4 sprigs flat-leaf parsley plus 2 tablespoons chopped parsley

2 sprigs thyme

¼ cup chopped celery leaves

1 bay leaf

¼ cup oil-packed sun-dried tomatoes

6 ounces silken soft tofu

¼ cup Dairy Milk Alternative (page 173)

1 clove garlic, minced

Salt

Freshly ground black pepper

Combine the wine, vinegar, lemon juice, peppercorns, parsley and thyme sprigs, celery leaves, and bay leaf in a small saucepan over high heat. Boil the liquid until it is reduced to ¼ cup, about 10 minutes. Strain the liquid through a fine-mesh sieve into a small bowl, and discard the solids.

Combine the sun-dried tomatoes, tofu, milk, garlic, chopped parsley, and wine mixture in a blender. Puree the mixture at top speed, occasionally scraping down the sides of the blender with a spatula, until smooth, about 1 minute. Return the mixture to the same saucepan and simmer over medium-low heat, stirring occasionally, for about 3 minutes to allow the flavors to fully blend. If a thinner sauce is desired, whisk in additional milk, 1 tablespoon at a time. Taste and correct the seasonings with salt and freshly ground black pepper. Serve warm.

spicy peanut sauce

Free of EGG SUGAR

MAKES 2 CUPS

This lively sauce combines rich sesame oil and date syrup with minced ginger, giving it a refreshing finish. Select a creamy-style peanut butter for this recipe, with little or no added sugar or salt. If you are using an old-fashioned peanut butter, in which the oil rises to the surface, be sure to mix the oil back in thoroughly before adding it to this recipe, or the sauce will separate once it cools.

1 cup smooth peanut butter

1/2 cup boiling water (more if needed)

3 tablespoons toasted sesame oil

3 tablespoons Date Syrup (page 189) or honey

2 tablespoons gluten-free tamari

2 tablespoons rice vinegar

3 cloves garlic, minced

1 tablespoon peeled, minced fresh ginger

1/8 teaspoon crushed red pepper flakes, or to taste

Combine the peanut butter and water in a bowl and stir until smooth. Add the sesame oil, date syrup, tamari, vinegar, garlic, ginger, and pepper flakes. Stir until well blended and smooth. To thin or rewarm the sauce, slowly stir in boiling water, a little at a time, until the desired consistency is achieved. Do not reheat it in a saucepan or in the microwave, or the sauce will break. Serve at room temperature.

mustard cream sauce

Free of EGG SOY NUT SUGAR OIL

MAKES 1 CUP

$^3/_4$ cup Vegetable Stock (page 177)

$^1/_3$ cup Dairy Milk Alternative (page 173)

$^1/_4$ cup dry white wine

2 tablespoons gluten-free Dijon mustard

1 tablespoon Date Syrup (page 189) or honey

1 tablespoon Gluten-Free Flour Mix (page 172)

1 teaspoon apple cider vinegar

2 teaspoons chopped fresh tarragon, or
$^1/_4$ teaspoon dried

In a blender combine the vegetable stock, milk, wine, mustard, date syrup, flour, and vinegar. Cover the blender and whirl at top speed for about 30 seconds to blend. Pour the mixture into a saucepan, add the tarragon, and cook over medium-high heat, whisking constantly, until the sauce begins to thicken, 5 to 6 minutes. If a thinner sauce is desired, whisk in an additional $^1/_4$ cup of milk. Serve hot.

mushroom sauce

Free of EGG SOY NUT SUGAR OIL

MAKES 2$^1/_2$ CUPS

1 cup Dairy Milk Alternative (page 173)

1 tablespoon Gluten-Free Flour Mix (page 172)

$^1/_2$ teaspoon sea salt

$^1/_8$ teaspoon ground white pepper

$^3/_4$ pound fresh button mushrooms, thinly sliced

1 tablespoon cream sherry

In a blender combine the milk, flour, salt, and pepper. Cover the blender and whirl at top speed for about 30 seconds to blend. Pour the mixture into a large saucepan and cook over medium heat, whisking constantly, until the sauce begins to thicken, about 3 to 4 minutes. Add the mushrooms, cover, and continue simmering, stirring occasionally, until the mixture is reduced by half, 6 to 7 minutes. Add the sherry and stir to blend. Serve hot.

lean sour cream

Free of EGG NUT SUGAR OIL

MAKES 1³/₄ CUPS

Even though sour cream may no longer be a part of my diet, I still want it on my baked potato. This soy version satisfies my craving and has all the flavor—without all the fat—of conventional dairy sour cream. In a pinch, you can also make sour cream by combining 1 (6-ounce) container of plain dairy-free yogurt with 1 teaspoon apple cider vinegar.

---

1 (12-ounce) package silken soft tofu, drained

¹/₄ cup Dairy Milk Alternative (page 173)

1 tablespoon freshly squeezed lemon juice

1 tablespoon apple cider vinegar

¹/₄ teaspoon salt

Combine the tofu, milk, lemon juice, vinegar, and salt in a blender. Puree the mixture at top speed, occasionally scraping down the sides of the blender with a spatula, until smooth, about 1 minute. Transfer the mixture to a container with a tight-fitting lid. The sour cream will keep, covered and refrigerated, for 2 days. Serve chilled, stirring with a spoon before serving.

pico de gallo

Free of EGG SOY NUT SUGAR OIL

MAKES 1¹/₂ CUPS

1 pound ripe tomatoes, seeded and diced

¹/₂ cup finely chopped red onion (about ¹/₂ small onion)

1/4 cup finely chopped fresh cilantro or flat-leaf parsley

2 tablespoons freshly squeezed lime juice (about 2 limes)

2 cloves garlic, minced

1 jalapeño pepper, seeded and minced, more or less to taste

¹/₄ teaspoon salt

¹/₈ teaspoon freshly ground black pepper

Combine the tomato, onion, cilantro, lime juice, garlic, jalapeño, salt, and pepper in a nonmetallic bowl, and toss to combine. Taste and correct the seasonings. Serve immediately, or cover the bowl tightly and refrigerate for up to 2 days. Just before serving, gently toss the salsa to mix. Serve chilled or at room temperature.

chunky guacamole

Free of EGG SOY NUT SUGAR OIL

MAKES 1¹/₂ CUPS

2 ripe avocados, 1 mashed and 1 diced

¹/₄ cup finely chopped red onion

2 cloves garlic, minced

1 medium tomato, diced

2 tablespoons lime juice (about 2 limes)

¹/₄ teaspoon salt

Combing the mashed avocado, onion, garlic, tomato, lime juice, and salt in a nonmetallic bowl, stirring to blend. Gently fold in the chopped avocado. Serve immediately or cover the bowl tightly and refrigerate for up to 3 hours. Serve chilled or at room temperature.

kiwi-papaya salsa

Free of EGG SOY NUT SUGAR OIL

MAKES 3 CUPS

1 cup peeled, diced kiwifruit, cut into ¼-inch pieces (3 to 4 kiwifruit)

1½ cups peeled, seeded, and diced ripe papaya, cut into ¼-inch pieces (about 1 large papaya)

⅓ cup minced chives (2 to 3 bunches)

2 ripe plum tomatoes, seeded and diced

2 teaspoons freshly squeezed lime juice

1 teaspoon grated lime zest

¼ teaspoon salt

⅛ teaspoon freshly ground black pepper

⅓ cup finely chopped flat-leaf parsley

Combine the kiwifruit, papaya, chives, tomato, lime juice, zest, salt, and pepper in a nonmetallic bowl and toss to mix. Cover the bowl tightly and refrigerate for up to 2 hours. Just before serving, add the parsley and toss gently to mix. Taste and correct the seasonings. Serve chilled.

edamame nut pâté

Free of EGG SUGAR OIL

SERVES 4

1¼ cups frozen shelled edamame, thawed

½ cup nut milk pulp (see page 173) or almond meal flour

1 cup mint, basil, or cilantro leaves (packed)

1 green onion, white and green parts, chopped

1 clove garlic

½ teaspoon salt

3 tablespoons freshly squeezed lemon juice or apple cider vinegar

3 tablespoons water (more if desired)

Combine the edamame, nut pulp, mint, green onion, garlic, and salt in a food processor or high-speed blender. Pulse the mixture several times until the edamame is coarsely chopped. With the motor running, add the lemon juice and water and continue to process until almost smooth but still has some texture. If serving as a dip, add more water, 1 tablespoon at a time, for the desired consistency. Transfer to a serving bowl, cover, and let stand until the flavors meld, at least 30 minutes, or refrigerate for up to 2 days.

zesty lemon hummus

Free of EGG SOY NUT SUGAR OIL

MAKES 2 CUPS

Whipping up a batch of hummus is amazingly simple to do and is a staple in our home. This protein powerhouse is versatile as a dip or a nutritious vegetarian sandwich spread. It's also easily adaptable. To make pesto hummus, simply add ¼ cup of Basil Pesto (page 129)

2 cups cooked chickpeas (see page 180), or 1 (15-ounce) can, drained and rinsed

⅓ cup tahini

¼ cup water

Zest of 1 lemon

3 tablespoon freshly squeezed lemon juice (about 1 lemon)

3 cloves garlic

1 tablespoon apple cider vinegar

¼ teaspoon ground cumin

¼ teaspoon salt

In a food processor or high-speed blender, combine the chickpeas, tahini, water, lemon zest, lemon juice, garlic, vinegar, cumin, and salt. Process the mixture, scraping down the sides with a rubber spatula as needed, until the hummus is smooth and creamy, about 3 minutes.

Transfer the hummus to a serving bowl, cover, and let stand until the flavors meld, at least 30 minutes, or refrigerate for up to 5 days. Allow the hummus to reach room temperature before serving and serve with gluten- and dairy-free crackers or vegetable crudités.

basil pesto

Free of EGG SOY SUGAR

MAKES 2¹/₂ CUPS

Pesto is so easy to makes and a delicious addition to pasta, pizza, soups, and hummus. Adding a little powdered vitamin C will help the pesto retain its bright green color. This recipe can easily be doubled, and by freezing it in ¹/₂-cup muffin tins, you can easily portion out exactly what you need.

2 cups whole fresh basil leaves, stemmed and tightly packed

¹/₃ cup pine nuts or walnut pieces

¹/₄ cup olive oil

3 cloves garlic

¹/₂ teaspoon sea salt

¹/₂ teaspoon powdered vitamin C, or 1 teaspoon lemon juice (optional)

Set aside a standard ¹/₂-cup muffin tin and plastic wrap.

TO PREPARE THE PESTO: In a food processor or high-speed blender, combine the basil, nuts, olive oil, garlic, salt, and vitamin C. Process the mixture, scraping down the sides with a rubber spatula as needed, until the pesto is smooth and creamy, about 3 minutes. Spoon the mixture into the muffin tins, cover with plastic wrap, and freeze overnight.

TO UNMOLD AND STORE THE PESTO: Tear off 6 sheets of plastic wrap and place them side-by-side on the counter. Run the back of the tin under hot tap water to release the molds. Using a rubber spatula, scoop each portion of frozen pesto onto 1 sheet of plastic; wrap tightly, store in a freezer bag, and freeze until ready to use. Frozen, this pesto will keep for 6 months.

olive anchovy tapenade

Free of EGG* SOY NUT SUGAR

MAKES 2 CUPS

This tapenade is a staple in our home. In addition to using it as a spread on gluten-free crackers and Aramanth Sesame Breadsticks (page 143), we've been known to add a spoonful to pasta sauce and salad dressings and to use it on sandwiches in place of mayonnaise. It's easy to make and will keep for up to 2 weeks when tightly covered in the refrigerator. If you're not fond of anchovies and choose to omit them, you'll still have a wonderful tapenade.

1 tablespoon olive oil (or steam-sauté, see page 18)

1 medium yellow onion, finely chopped

2 cloves garlic, minced

$1/2$ cup pitted, minced kalamata olives or other brine-cured black olives

$1/2$ cup pitted, minced green olives

4 canned anchovy fillets, minced

2 tablespoons finely chopped pimiento

1 tablespoon freshly squeezed lemon juice

$1/4$ teaspoon freshly ground black pepper

$1/4$ cup minced fresh basil leaves

2 tablespoons capers, drained

Toasted Three Seed Bread* (page 138) or dairy- and gluten-free crackers, for serving

TO PREPARE THE TAPENADE: Heat the olive oil in a skillet over medium-high heat and sauté the onion until tender, about 3 minutes. Add the garlic and sauté for about 30 seconds. Remove from the heat and allow the mixture to cool slightly.

Combine the olives, anchovies, pimiento, lemon juice, pepper, and cooled onion mixture in a container with a tight-fitting lid; use a rubber spatula to blend the mixture thoroughly. Gently stir in the basil and capers until just incorporated. Cover and refrigerate.

TO SERVE THE SPREAD: Remove the tapenade from the refrigerator and allow it to reach room temperature. Serve the tapenade with toasted Three Seed Bread or gluten-free crackers.

eggplant-sesame-basil spread

Free of EGG* SOY NUT SUGAR

MAKES ABOUT 2¹/₂ CUPS

Although the eggplant can be broiled, grilling it on the barbecue imparts a wonderful smoky flavor that pairs nicely with the nutty toasted sesame seeds.

---

2 pounds Japanese or globe eggplant, peeled and sliced 1 inch thick

Salt, for salting eggplant

¹/₃ cup olive oil, plus more for brushing

1 cup chopped green onion, white and green parts (about 1 bunch)

3 cloves garlic, minced

¹/₄ cup chopped fresh basil

1 large, ripe tomato, peeled and quartered, with juices (see page 179)

1 tablespoon freshly squeezed lemon juice

1 teaspoon Date Syrup (page 189)

¹/₂ teaspoon sea salt

¹/₄ teaspoon freshly ground black pepper

2 teaspoons toasted sesame oil

1 tablespoon sesame seeds, toasted (see page 186)

Herb Toast* (page 185) or gluten-free crackers, for serving

TO PREPARE THE EGGPLANT: With a knife, score the eggplant slices diagonally 5 or 6 times about

¹/₂-inch deep, and sprinkle both sides with salt. Line a colander with paper towel and transfer the eggplant to the colander to drain for about 45 minutes. Using fresh paper towels, dry the eggplant by patting it with the towels and brush away any remaining salt.

Preheat the broiler and position the rack about 6 inches from the heat source. Generously brush the eggplant with olive oil. Place the eggplant on a broiler pan, cut-side up, and broil for 8 to 10 minutes. With tongs, turn the eggplant over and continue broiling until it is very soft, 8 to 10 minutes longer. Transfer the eggplant to a plate to cool for about 15 minutes.

TO PREPARE THE SPREAD: Heat 1 tablespoon of the olive oil in a small skillet over medium-high heat. Sauté the onion, garlic, and basil until the onion is softened, about 1 minute. Remove from the heat and set aside.

When the eggplant is cool enough to handle, cut it into 2-inch pieces. Combine with the tomato, remaining olive oil (about ¹/₄ cup), lemon juice, date syrup, salt, and pepper in a blender. Pulse about 10 times. The mixture should be slightly chunky. Stir in the onion mixture and the sesame oil and season to taste. To serve, stir in half of the sesame seeds and sprinkle the rest on top.

caramelized balsamic onions *with* mushrooms

Free of EGG* SOY NUT SUGAR OIL

MAKES 3 CUPS

Caramelizing the onions and mushrooms allows their flavors to mingle and is well worth the time involved. This recipe is made without the use of oil, but if you prefer a Mediterranean classic, simply omit the vegetable stock and sauté the mixture with 2 tablespoons of olive oil instead. Serve as a spread, or for a robust vegetable dish, toss with tender cooked green beans. It also makes a flavorful topping for a Spanish Tortilla (page 35).

2 large yellow onions, very thinly sliced

2 medium red onions, very thinly sliced

1/4 pound fresh button mushrooms, thinly sliced

1/4 cup Vegetable Stock (page 177), or more if needed

1/2 teaspoon Date Syrup (page 189) or honey

5 sprigs thyme

1/2 teaspoon salt

1/8 teaspoon freshly ground black pepper

3 tablespoons balsamic vinegar

2 cloves garlic, minced

Toasted Three Seed Bread* (page 138) or dairy- and gluten-free crackers as accompaniment

TO PREPARE THE SPREAD: Heat a large skillet over medium-low heat and add the onions, mushrooms, stock, date syrup, thyme, salt, and pepper. Stir to combine. Cover and cook the mixture, stirring occasionally, about 20 minutes. Remove the lid and add the vinegar and garlic. Stir to blend. Continue cooking, uncovered, until most of the liquid has evaporated and the onions have caramelized, 45 to 55 minutes. If the mixture begins to stick to the bottom of the pan, add additional stock 1 tablespoon at a time. Remove the thyme sprigs and season to taste. Serve immediately or allow the spread to reach room temperature; cover and refrigerate for up to 5 days. Before serving, warm it in a small saucepan at low heat, stirring occasionally, about 5 minutes.

summer's harvest ratatouille

Free of EGG SOY NUT SUGAR OIL

MAKES 5 TO 6 CUPS

My Tete (Aunt) Danie's ratatouille is at the top of our family's list of adored foods. She used to prepare it from the summer bounty of vine-ripened tomatoes and vegetables from my uncle's garden and then can it, so that we could enjoy the taste of summer during the winter months. I remember it fondly, as it always graced her holiday table as part of the antipasto platter.

2 red onions, coarsely chopped

2 pounds Japanese or globe eggplant, unpeeled, cut into 1-inch pieces

1 large red bell pepper, seeded, ribbed, and cut into 1-inch pieces

1 large yellow bell pepper, seeded, ribbed, and cut into 1-inch pieces

4 cloves garlic, minced

$1/2$ teaspoon sea salt

$1/4$ teaspoon freshly ground black pepper

$1/4$ cup water

1 pound zucchini, halved lengthwise and cut into 1-inch pieces

2 pounds ripe tomatoes, seeded and coarsely chopped (about 3 cups)

2 teaspoons coriander seeds

3 sprigs thyme

1 teaspoon minced fresh rosemary

1 bay leaf

$1/4$ cup minced flat-leaf parsley

1 tablespoon freshly squeezed lemon juice

In a large sauté pan over medium-high heat add the onion, eggplant, peppers, garlic, salt, pepper, and water. Sauté the mixture until tender and the liquid has evaporated, about 10 minutes, stirring occasionally. Add the zucchini, tomato, coriander, thyme, rosemary, and bay leaf, and sauté until blended, 2 to 3 minutes. Cover, decrease the heat to medium-low, and simmer, stirring occasionally, until the vegetables are tender, about 20 minutes. Remove from the heat, add the parsley and lemon, and toss to incorporate. Remove the bay leaf and thyme sprigs, taste, and correct the seasonings. Transfer the ratatouille to a bowl and allow to cool. Cover and refrigerate. Serve cold, warm, or hot. It can be made 2 days ahead.

apple mango chutney

Free of EGG SOY NUT SUGAR OIL

MAKES 2 CUPS

1³/₄ pounds pippin or Granny Smith apples, peeled, cored, and minced

1 ripe mango, peeled, pitted, and cut into ¹/₂-inch pieces

1 large yellow onion, finely chopped

¹/₃ cup golden raisins

¹/₄ cup red wine vinegar

¹/₂ teaspoon freshly squeezed lemon juice

¹/₄ cup Date Syrup (page 189)

1 tablespoon peeled, minced fresh ginger, or 1 teaspoon ground

¹/₂ teaspoon ground turmeric

¹/₈ teaspoon sea salt

Pinch of crushed red pepper flakes

Combine all the ingredients in a large saucepan over medium-high heat and stir to blend. Bring to a boil. Cover, cracking the lid to allow steam to escape, and decrease the heat to low. Simmer for about 1 hour, stirring occasionally. Remove from the heat and allow the mixture to cool for about 2 hours. Transfer to a container with a tight-fitting lid and refrigerate. Stir before serving and allow it to reach room temperature.

applesauce

Free of EGG SOY NUT SUGAR OIL

MAKES 4 CUPS

1¹/₂ pounds Granny Smith or pippin apples, peeled, cored, and sliced

1¹/₂ pounds Gala or McIntosh apples, peeled, cored, and sliced

¹/₂ cup water

1 tablespoon Date Syrup (page 189), or to taste

1 tablespoon freshly squeezed lemon juice

Combine the apples and water in a large sauce-pan over medium-low heat. Cover and cook until the apples are very soft, about 20 minutes, stirring occasionally. Transfer to a bowl and mash with a fork or potato masher. Add the date syrup and lemon juice to taste, depending. Serve warm or at room temperature. To store, cover and refrigerate for up to 1 week

yeasted and quick breads

My father always loved bread, and in fact made his living working for a bakery. When I was a little girl, he often took me for rides in his delivery truck—the intoxicating aroma of the freshly baked goods along with the treasured moments shared with my dad made my heart soar. So when gluten in my diet was no longer an option, the thought of giving up bread was initially devastating. But I was determined to discover new ingredients and techniques that would allow me to eat the breads I love. Here are my favorites—enjoy!

GLUTEN-FREE BAKING TIPS

- **Oven temperature matters:** Double check your oven temperature with an oven thermometer to determine if your oven is a slow or fast oven, and adjust cooking times accordingly.

- **Measuring:** Unlike savory cooking, where the chef can add a little more of this or that to customize a recipe, baking requires more accuracy; this is especially true with alternative flours and liquids. It's important to use dry measuring cups for dry ingredients—always leveling them off. The same holds true for measuring spoons, and for liquids, use a leveled liquid measuring cup.

- **Instant-read thermometer:** Several of the bread recipes will require an internal temperature reading. The difference between a perfectly baked loaf of gluten-free bread and one that is slightly underdone can be as little as 5 degrees.

- **Parchment paper:** I've reduced the unnecessary fats in many of the recipes, so for effortless release of your baked goods, parchment paper is indispensable.

- **Bring all ingredients to room temperature:** this is particularly important with yeasted bread recipes.

- **Proofing yeasted bread:** A warm, not hot, (90°F to 115°F) location away from drafts with humidity of about 80 percent is the most desirable condition to allow yeasted doughs and batters to rise. During the summer this is easily achieved; however, during the winter it can be a bit more challenging. A method I like to use is called "oven proofing," and this is how it works: Preheat the oven to 150°F. Cover the prepared dough with a damp towel loosely covering the pan, place the pan in the oven, close the door, and immediately turn off the heat. Allow the dough or batter to rise for the allotted time, and then bake as directed. Be sure to check the date on the yeast packaging; the yeast must be fresh for the bread to rise. To keep it fresh, store it in the refrigerator until ready to use.

fiber-rich sandwich bread

Free of SOY NUT SUGAR OIL

MAKES 1 LOAF

This sandwich loaf is absolutely divine. If you hadn't baked it yourself you would never believe it was gluten- and dairy-free. It's light and airy, has a good dose of fiber from the flax and dates, and does not contain any refined sweeteners or oil.

---

3 cups Gluten-Free Flour Mix (page 172)

2 teaspoons xanthan gum

2 tablespoons ground flax meal

1 tablespoon active dry yeast

$^1/_2$ teaspoon salt

2 large eggs

$^1/_2$ cup Dairy Milk Alternative (page 173)

$^1/_2$ cup water

$^1/_4$ cup Date Syrup (page 189) or honey

1 teaspoon apple cider vinegar

Coat an $8^1/_2$ by $4^1/_2$-inch bread pan with cooking spray and line with parchment paper. Set aside.

TO PREPARE THE DOUGH: Combine the flour, xanthan gum, flax, yeast, and salt in a bowl. Mix together with a whisk until thoroughly blended; set aside.

Using a hand mixer set on medium speed, beat the eggs in a large bowl until blended. In a small saucepan, whisk the milk, water, date syrup, and vinegar until blended. Heat the mixture over medium-low heat, until warm but not hot, 110°F to 115°F. Pour the milk mixture into the egg and beat until just foamy. Gradually add the flour mixture to the bowl and beat until combined, scraping down the sides as needed.

TO BAKE THE BREAD: Spoon the batter into the prepared pan and smooth out the top with the back of an oiled spoon. Cover the pan with a damp kitchen towel and place it in a warm, draft free location for 50 to 60 minutes or until the dough crests just above the top of the pan. Meanwhile, position the rack in the center of the oven and preheat the oven to 350°F.

Place the pan in the center of the preheated oven and bake for 50 minutes, or until an instant-read thermometer inserted into the center of the loaf, without touching the bottom of the pan, reads 206°F to 208°F. Remove the pan from the oven and turn the bread out of the pan. Discard the parchment paper and place the loaf back in the oven, directly on the oven rack, and bake for 5 minutes longer. Transfer the bread to a wire rack and cool completely before slicing.

three seed bread

MAKES ONE 9-INCH LOAF

This protein-packed, seeded quick bread is loaded with vitamins, minerals, and fiber. It serves as a delicious accompaniment to any savory dish. This is the bread for those who cannot tolerate yeasted breads, and it can be used as a replacement in any of the recipes calling for Fiber-Rich Sandwich bread.

1 cup plain unsweetened soy yogurt

2 large eggs

1 teaspoon apple cider vinegar

1 tablespoon raw sunflower seeds

1 tablespoon raw pumpkin seeds

2 cups Gluten-Free Flour Mix (page 172)

2 teaspoons gluten-free baking powder

1/2 teaspoon baking soda

1 tablespoon whole flax seed

1/2 teaspoon salt

Preheat the oven to 350°F. Lightly grease an 8¹/₂ by 4¹/₂ by 2¹/₂-inch loaf pan with a small amount of oil. Sprinkle the bottom of the pan with 1 tablespoon each of the sunflower and pumpkin seeds. Set aside.

TO PREPARE THE BATTER: Whisk the yogurt, eggs, and vinegar together in a large bowl. Set aside. Combine the flour, baking powder, baking soda, flax seed, and salt in a bowl. In a spice grinder or food processor, coarsely grind the remaining 2 tablespoons of sunflower and pumpkin seeds. Add the ground seeds to the flour mixture and whisk until well blended. Pour the yogurt mixture into the flour mixture and mix until just combined. Do not overmix the batter.

TO BAKE THE BREAD: Pour the batter into the prepared loaf pan and smooth out the batter as much as possible. Bake the bread until lightly browned, about 50 minutes, or until the internal temperature reaches 206°F on an instant-read thermometer. Allow the loaf to cool 15 minutes in the pan, then turn it out onto a wire rack to cool completely, about 1 hour. Once cool, place the loaf on a cutting board and, using a serrated bread knife, slice it into ³/₄-inch-thick pieces. Store the slices by wrapping each piece in plastic wrap and placing them in an airtight container for up to 5 days, or freeze for up to 2 weeks.

orange popovers

Free of SOY SUGAR OIL

MAKES 10 TO 12 POPOVERS

These delicate, fragile shells puff as they bake, creating air pockets that can be filled with preserves or with a savory stew. Once the popovers are in the oven, resist the temptation to open the oven door for a peek. As the popovers begin to rise above the lip of the cup, the slightest draft will cause them to fall. I've tested this recipe with dairy milk alternatives, including coconut beverages, and the results were disappointing; stick with the light coconut milk, it works beautifully!

1 cup Gluten-Free Flour Mix (page 172)

1 tablespoon chopped orange zest (about 2 oranges)

¼ teaspoon xanthan gum

¼ teaspoon salt

4 large eggs

1 cup canned light coconut milk, stirred

1 teaspoon Orange Date Syrup (page 189)

Position the rack in the center of the oven and preheat the oven to 450°F. Coat a muffin pan or popover pan with cooking spray and set aside.

TO PREPARE THE BATTER: Combine the flour, zest, xanthan gum, and salt in a large bowl. Mix together with a whisk. In a separate bowl with an electric mixer, beat the eggs, coconut milk, and date syrup, about 1 minute. Pour the coconut mixture into the flour mixture and beat to combine; the batter will be very runny. Pour the batter into the prepared muffin cups, filling each cup about two-thirds full. Bake the popovers for 15 minutes, then lower the oven temperature to 350°F and bake until the popovers are richly browned, about 25 minutes longer. Remove the popovers from the pan and serve hot.

NOTE: In place of the light coconut milk, you may also use unsweetened canned coconut milk in this recipe, but you will need to dilute it. First, thoroughly blend the coconut milk. Then, in a liquid measuring cup, combine ⅓ cup of the coconut milk and ⅔ cup of water; stir to blend.

crispy pizza crust

MAKES ONE 12-INCH ROUND

This cracker-like pizza crust is amazingly versatile, simple to assemble, and is made without the use of yeast or oil. Use this crust in the traditional sense as the base for the Rustic Heirloom Pesto Pizza (page 96) or the Rustic Mushroom Pizza (page 98) or as a flatbread cracker to accompany your favorite spread, such as Zesty Lemon Hummus (page 128), Caramelized Balsamic Onions with Mushrooms (page 132), or Eggplant-Sesame-Basil Spread (page 131).

1¹/₃ cup Gluten-Free Flour Mix (page 172)

2 teaspoons gluten-free baking powder

¹/₄ teaspoon xanthan gum

¹/₄ teaspoon dried thyme

¹/₄ teaspoon dried oregano

¹/₄ teaspoon garlic powder

¹/₄ teaspoon salt

1 cup water

Preheat the oven to 425°F. Line a metal pizza pan with parchment paper. Set aside.

TO PREPARE THE BATTER: Combine the flour, baking powder, xanthan gum, thyme, oregano, garlic powder, and salt in a large bowl. Thoroughly mix together with a whisk until fully combined. Add the water to the flour mixture, and with a rubber spatula stir to combine. Working quickly, pour the batter onto the parchment paper and smooth it out; the batter should be less than ¹/₂ inch thick. Pre-bake the crust for 15 minutes. Remove the crust from the oven and follow the directions for Rustic Mushroom Pizza (page 98) or Rustic Heirloom Pesto Pizza (page 96). If using this crust to make flatbread crackers, bake 5 to 8 minutes longer, until golden and crispy. Cool completely before breaking it up into random sized pieces, and serve with your favorite dip or spread.

traditional pizza crust

MAKES ONE 12-INCH ROUND

Thick or thin, it's your call with this traditional yeasted crust. For a thinner crust simply spread out the batter and bake the crust. For a loftier goal, allow the dough to rise for about 30 minutes before baking. Either way, this crust makes a delicious pizza. For a crispier crust, bake the dough on a pre-heated pizza stone.

³/₄ cup Dairy Milk Alternative (page 173), warmed to 110°F to 115°F

¹/₂ teaspoon Date Syrup (page 189)

1 package (2¹/₄ teaspoons) quick-rise dry yeast

1¹/₂ cups Gluten-Free Flour Mix (page 172)

1 teaspoon xanthan gum

¹/₂ teaspoon dried oregano

¹/₄ teaspoon dried thyme

¹/₄ teaspoon garlic powder

¹/₄ teaspoon salt

1 tablespoon olive oil

1 teaspoon apple cider vinegar

Preheat the oven to 425°F. Lightly spray a metal pizza pan with cooking spray and line it with parchment paper. Set aside.

TO PREPARE THE DOUGH: In a small bowl, combine the warm milk and date syrup; stir to blend. Add the yeast and stir until the yeast has dissolved, then set aside until the mixture has doubled in volume, about 10 minutes. Meanwhile, in a large bowl, add the flour, xanthan gum, oregano, thyme, garlic powder, and salt. Thoroughly mix together with a whisk until fully combined. Add the oil and vinegar to the milk mixture and stir to blend. Add the milk mixture to the flour mixture and, with a rubber spatula, stir to fully combine. Spoon the dough onto the prepared pan, smoothing out the center and, with wet hands, building up the edges slightly. Cover the dough with a damp kitchen towel and place it in a warm, draft-free location for about 20 minutes or until the dough has risen slightly. Bake the crust for 15 minutes. Remove the crust from the oven and follow recipe directions for Rustic Mushroom Pizza (page 98) or Rustic Heirloom Pesto Pizza (page 96).

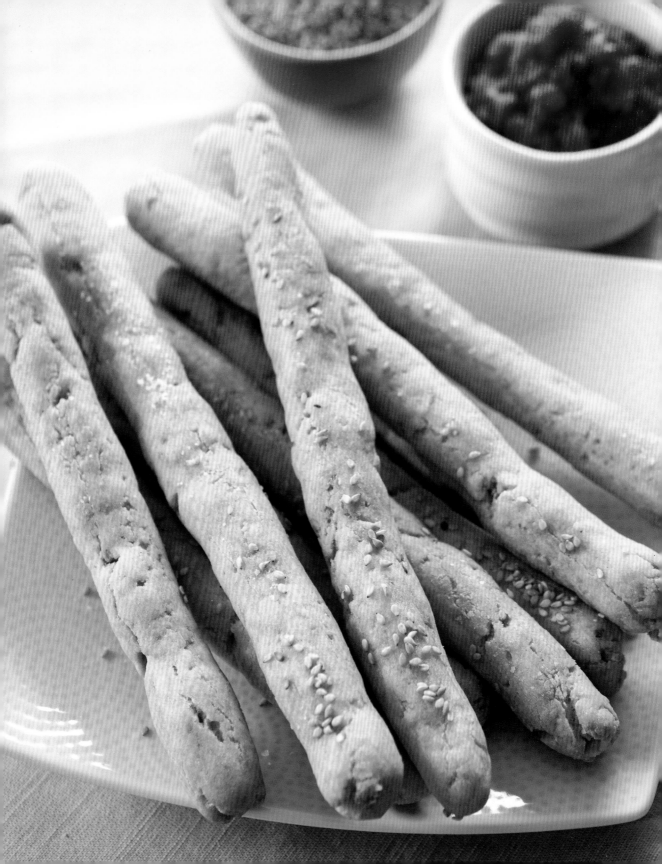

amaranth sesame breadsticks

Free of EGG SOY NUT

MAKES 12 BREADSTICKS

Not too hard and not too soft, but just right. These breadsticks are fun to make and particularly good with soup, salad, and dips. Serve them hot from the oven, but be warned; they'll disappear before you know it!

1 cup amaranth flour

¹/₂ cup Gluten-Free Flour Mix (page 172)

1 tablespoon toasted sesame seeds, plus more for sprinkling

1 tablespoon sugar

1 teaspoon xanthan gum

¹/₂ teaspoon salt

¹/₂ teaspoon onion powder

³/₄ cup warm water (110°F to 115°F)

1 package (2¹/₄ teaspoons) quick-rise dry yeast

1 teaspoon olive oil

Kosher salt, for sprinkling (optional)

Position the rack in the center of the oven and preheat to 400°F. Lightly coat a baking sheet with cooking spray and line with parchment paper. Set aside.

TO PREPARE THE DOUGH: Combine the amaranth flour, flour, sesame seeds, sugar, xanthan gum, salt, and onion powder in a large bowl. Mix together with a whisk until blended. In a small bowl dissolve the yeast in warm water and whisk in the olive oil. Pour the yeast mixture into the flour mixture. Using a sturdy wooden spoon, stir until the mixture comes together and forms a ball. Divide the dough into 12 balls. Line a flat work surface with parchment or waxed paper. Using your hands, roll the dough to form 12-inch-long, cigar-shaped rolls. Transfer the rolls to the prepared pan. Cover the pan with a damp kitchen towel and place it in a warm, draft-free location for 20 minutes or until the breadsticks have risen slightly. If desired, sprinkle with kosher salt. Place the pan in the preheated oven and bake for 20 minutes, or until the breadsticks are dark golden brown and slightly crisp on the bottom. If desired, sprinkle with additional sesame seeds.

rosemary drop biscuits

Free of EGG SOY NUT SUGAR

MAKES 10 BISCUITS

These biscuits lend themselves nicely to stews and hearty soups. Deliciously enveloped in rosemary essence, they are tender on the inside and slightly crusty on the outside. For a comforting autumn meal, serve them alongside Shepherd's Pie (page 88). To easily portion the batter, I like using a ¼-cup (#16) ice cream scoop, available at most cooking stores and restaurant suppliers.

1 cup Dairy Milk Alternative (page 173)

1 tablespoon apple cider vinegar

2 cups Gluten-Free Flour Mix (page 172)

1 tablespoon minced fresh rosemary

2 teaspoons gluten-free baking powder

½ teaspoon baking soda

½ teaspoon xanthan gum

½ teaspoon salt

3 tablespoons coconut oil or dairy-free margarine

Preheat the oven to 450°F. Line an insulated baking sheet with parchment paper.

TO PREPARE THE DOUGH: Combine the milk and vinegar in a measuring cup, stir to blend, and set aside. Combine the flour, rosemary, baking powder, baking soda, xanthan gum, and salt in a large bowl. Whisk until thoroughly blended. Add the coconut oil and crumble the mixture with your fingertips until it resembles coarse pebbles. Add the milk to the flour mixture and stir with a rubber spatula until just incorporated and the batter pulls away from the sides of the bowl.

TO FORM AND BAKE THE BISCUITS: Using a greased ¼-cup measuring cup, scoop a level amount of batter and drop it onto the prepared baking sheet. Repeat with the remaining batter, placing the biscuits about 2 inches apart. Bake until golden brown, 16 to 18 minutes. Serve warm.

sweet potato cornbread

Free of SOY NUT SUGAR OIL

SERVES 4 TO 6

*Moist with just a hint of sweetness, this easy corn-
bread is a great companion for Blackstrap Beans
(page 104) or anytime you need to whip up a quick
bread to accompany a meal.*

1 cup Gluten-Free Flour Mix (page 172)

1 cup yellow fine or medium ground cornmeal

2¹/₂ teaspoons gluten-free baking powder

¹/₂ teaspoon xanthan gum

¹/₂ teaspoon salt

2 large eggs

¹/₂ cup Dairy Milk Alternative (page 173)

¹/₂ cup Orange Date Syrup (page 189)

1 cup baked, peeled, and mashed ruby yam
(about 1 medium yam)

¹/₂ cup white corn kernels, fresh (about 1 ear)
or frozen

Preheat the oven to 400°F. Lightly grease an 8 by
8 by 2-inch glass baking dish with olive oil.

TO PREPARE THE BATTER: Combine the flour, cornmeal, baking powder, xanthan gum, and salt in
a large bowl. Mix together with a whisk and set
aside.

Whisk the eggs, milk, and date syrup together
in a bowl. Add the yam and corn, mixing until
well blended. Pour the egg mixture into the flour
mixture and mix until just combined. Do not
overmix, as this can cause the cornbread to be
tough.

TO BAKE THE BREAD: Pour the batter into the prepared baking dish and bake until firm and lightly
browned, about 35 minutes. Allow the bread
to cool slightly, about 15 minutes, slice into
squares, and serve warm in the baking dish.

maple raisin scones

Free of EGG SOY* NUT SUGAR

MAKES 8 SCONES

My husband loves these scones warm out of the oven; they have a fine, tender crumb and a rich yet delicate maple flavor. The secret to having a tender crumb is in working the chilled margarine into the flour; once incorporated, the pieces of margarine should be the size of peas. These scones are amazingly easy to make and are a special addition to breakfast, brunch, or high tea.

$^{1}/_{2}$ **cup plain dairy-free yogurt***

$^{1}/_{4}$ **cup pure maple syrup**

$^{1}/_{4}$ **cup plus 2 tablespoons Date Syrup (page 189)**

1 cup raisins, golden raisins, or currants

3 cups Gluten-Free Flour Mix (page 172)

1$^{1}/_{2}$ teaspoons gluten-free baking powder

1 teaspoon xanthan gum

$^{1}/_{2}$ **teaspoon baking soda**

$^{1}/_{4}$ **teaspoon sea salt**

$^{1}/_{2}$ **cup dairy-free margarine*, cut into 1-inch pieces**

Preheat the oven to 375°F. Line an insulated baking sheet with parchment paper.

TO PREPARE THE DOUGH: Whisk together the yogurt, maple syrup, and the $^{1}/_{4}$ cup of date syrup in a small bowl. Stir in the raisins and set aside.

Combine the flour, baking powder, xanthan gum, baking soda, and salt in a large bowl and mix together with a whisk. Add the margarine and crumble the mixture through your fingertips until it resembles coarse pebbles. Add the liquid ingredients to the flour mixture and stir until the dough starts to come together. Using your hands, fold the dough over in the bowl 5 or 6 times, being careful not to overwork the dough; the dough will be slightly sticky.

TO FORM AND BAKE THE SCONES: Turn the dough out onto a lightly floured surface. Using your hands, pat out and shape the dough to form an 8-inch round. Cut the round evenly into 8 wedges. Using a metal spatula, transfer the wedges to the prepared baking sheet, about 1 inch apart. Using a pastry brush, lightly coat the wedges with the remaining 2 tablespoons of the date syrup.

Bake the scones until the tops are golden brown, about 20 minutes. Serve warm, or allow to cool completely on a wire rack, about 35 minutes, before storing in an airtight container.

lemon poppyseed muffins

Free of SOY NUT

MAKES 10 MUFFINS

These fragrant muffins have a tart, refreshing taste of lemon, complemented by a delightful light crunch from the poppyseeds. Ginger lovers can easily adapt this recipe to make Lemon Ginger Muffins by substituting 3 tablespoons of peeled, grated fresh ginger for the poppyseeds.

2 cups Gluten-Free Flour Mix (page 172)

1 tablespoon gluten-free baking powder

1/2 teaspoon baking soda

1/4 teaspoon salt

1/3 cup sugar

2 tablespoons poppyseeds

2 large eggs

1 cup Dairy Milk Alternative (page 173)

1 tablespoon freshly squeezed lemon juice

1/4 cup canola oil

2 tablespoons chopped lemon zest (from 3 to 4 lemons)

Position the rack in the center of the oven and preheat the oven to 400°F. Coat a muffin pan with cooking spray and set aside.

TO PREPARE THE BATTER: Combine the flour, baking powder, baking soda, salt, sugar, and poppyseeds in a large bowl. Mix together with a whisk until blended. Whisk together the eggs, milk, lemon juice, oil, and zest in a small bowl until well blended. Stir the egg mixture into the flour mixture until just combined, taking care not to overmix the batter. The batter should look lumpy.

TO BAKE THE MUFFINS: Spoon the batter into the prepared muffin tins, filling each cup two-thirds full. Any cups that are not filled with batter should be filled halfway with water to allow for even baking. Bake until golden brown and a tester inserted into the center comes out clean, about 20 minutes. Remove the pan from the oven and let cool for about 10 minutes. Transfer the muffins to a wire rack and cool completely.

blueberry corn muffins

Free of SOY NUT

MAKES 12 MUFFINS

For an exceptional treat, these muffins, with their moist, light, and tender crumb, brimming with blueberries, should be served warm from the oven while the juices are still bubbling. The turmeric enhances the color of the corn flour, providing a beautiful setting to showcase the blueberries.

1 cup Gluten-Free Flour Mix (page 172)

$^1/_2$ cup corn flour (Masa Harina)

$^1/_3$ cup granulated sugar

2$^1/_4$ teaspoons gluten-free baking powder

$^1/_2$ teaspoon baking soda

$^1/_4$ teaspoon turmeric

$^1/_4$ teaspoon xanthan gum

$^1/_4$ teaspoon salt

2 large eggs

$^1/_3$ cup unsweetened applesauce (see page 134)

$^1/_3$ cup unsweetened apple juice

3 tablespoons canola oil

1 teaspoon gluten-free vanilla extract

1 tablespoon freshly squeezed lemon juice

$^3/_4$ cup fresh blueberries, sorted, rinsed, and patted dry, or frozen (do not thaw)

Position the rack in the center of the oven and preheat the oven to 350°F. Lightly coat a muffin pan with cooking spray and set aside.

TO PREPARE THE BATTER: Combine the flours, sugar, baking powder, baking soda, turmeric, xanthan gum, and salt in a large bowl. Mix together with a whisk until well blended.

In a separate bowl, whisk together the eggs, applesauce, juice, oil, vanilla, and lemon juice until well blended. Stir the egg mixture into the flour mixture until just combined. Gently fold in the blueberries until just incorporated, taking care not to overmix the batter. The batter should look lumpy.

TO BAKE THE MUFFINS: Spoon the batter into the prepared muffin tins, filling each cup two-thirds full. Any cups that are not filled with batter should be filled halfway with water to allow for even baking. Bake the muffins until golden brown and a tester inserted in the center comes out clean, about 20 minutes. Remove the pan from the oven and let cool for about 5 minutes and serve warm. To store, transfer the muffins to a wire rack and cool completely before storing them in an airtight container.

cranberry-banana oat bread

Free of   SOY   NUT   SUGAR   OIL

MAKES ONE 9-INCH LOAF

With its moist, tender crumb and the sweet tang of cranberries, this quick bread is a staple at our Thanksgiving breakfast table. By adding your choice of chopped nuts or any type of dried fruit in place of the cranberries, you can easily adapt this basic recipe to your taste.

1¼ cups Gluten-Free Flour Mix (page 172)

¾ cup gluten-free quick oats

1 tablespoon gluten-free baking powder

½ teaspoon xanthan gum

½ teaspoon salt

2 large eggs

1 cup mashed ripe banana (about 2 medium bananas)

½ cup Date Syrup (page 189)

¼ teaspoon lemon juice or apple cider vinegar

⅓ cup dried cranberries

Preheat the oven to 350°F. Coat an 8½ by 4½-inch bread pan with cooking spray and line with parchment paper. Set aside.

TO PREPARE THE BATTER: Combine the flour, oats, baking powder, xanthan gum, and salt in a bowl. Thoroughly mix together with a whisk and set aside. Whisk the eggs, banana, date syrup, and lemon juice together in a large bowl. Add the cranberries and mix until blended. Stir in the flour mixture and mix until fully combined.

TO BAKE THE BREAD: Pour the batter into the prepared pan and with a rubber spatula, smooth out the top. Loosely cover the pan with aluminum foil (so that steam can escape), and bake for 35 minutes. Remove the foil and bake 25 minutes longer or until an instant-read thermometer inserted into the center of the loaf, without touching the bottom of the pan, reads 200°F. Allow the loaf to cool 10 minutes in the pan, then turn it out onto a wire rack, remove the parchment paper, and cool completely, about 1 hour. Using a serrated bread knife, slice the loaf into ¾-inch-thick pieces. Store the bread by wrapping each piece in plastic wrap and placing them in an airtight container for up to 5 days, or freeze for up to 2 weeks.

zucchini orange bread

Free of SOY SUGAR OIL

MAKES ONE 9-INCH LOAF

Fragrant orange zest paired with moist zucchini makes this quick bread a favorite with afternoon tea. The recipe is easy to prepare and is a great way to use up an abundance of zucchini from a summer garden. For a nice surprise, double the recipe and bake it in baby loaf pans to make homemade gifts for family and friends.

1½ cups Gluten-Free Flour Mix (page 172)

2 tablespoons ground flax meal

2 teaspoons gluten-free baking powder

½ teaspoon baking soda

½ teaspoon xanthan gum

¼ teaspoon salt

⅓ cup chopped pecans or walnuts

1 tablespoon grated orange zest (about 1 orange)

2 large eggs

½ cup orange Date Syrup (page 189)

1 cup grated zucchini (about 1 medium zucchini)

Preheat the oven to 350°F. Coat an 8½ by 4½-inch loaf pan with cooking spray and line with parchment paper. Set aside.

TO PREPARE THE BATTER: Combine the flour, flax meal, baking powder, baking soda, xanthan gum, and salt in a bowl. Mix together with a whisk. Add the nuts and zest and stir to combine; set aside.

Whisk the eggs and date syrup together in a large bowl. Grate the zucchini onto several layers of paper towel, place additional paper towel on top, and press out any excess moisture. Add the zucchini to the egg mixture and stir to blend. Gently stir the flour mixture into the zucchini mixture until just combined.

TO BAKE THE BREAD: Pour the batter into the prepared pan and with a rubber spatula, smooth out the top. Loosely cover the pan with aluminum foil (so that steam can escape), and bake for 35 minutes. Remove the foil and bake 25 minutes longer or until an instant-read thermometer inserted into the center of the loaf, without touching the bottom of the pan, reads 200°F. Allow the loaf to cool 10 minutes in the pan, then turn it out onto a wire rack to cool completely, about 1 hour. Using a serrated bread knife, slice the loaf into 3/4-inch-thick pieces. Store the bread by wrapping each piece in plastic wrap and placing them in an airtight container for up to 5 days, or freeze for up to 2 weeks.

sweet endings

I developed these recipes with the idea that dessert should still be a delicious and decadent treat you look forward to having once in a while. Several of the recipes such as the Lemon-Blueberry Tart (page 158), Spicy Ginger Cookies (page 166), or Cake Brownies with Orange Essence (page 169) are just some of the desserts that contain no refined sugar or oil, making them healthy alternatives to their dairy and fat cousins, but they're still desserts after all, so go easy.

bread pudding *with* pears *and* chocolate

Free of SOY* NUT OIL*

SERVES 6

It's hard to imagine improving on an old-fashioned comfort food like bread pudding. This version combines pears and chocolate and uses gluten-free bread and fresh Bosc pears. The result is a moist bread pudding with a soufflé-like texture.

6 cups cubed, lightly packed, day-old Fiber-Rich Sandwich Bread (page 137) or Three Seed Bread (page 138), cut into 1-inch pieces

2 Bosc pears, cored, peeled, and cut lengthwise into about 16 pieces

¼ cup dairy-free and gluten-free chocolate chips*

⅓ cup firmly packed light brown sugar

6 large eggs

3½ cups vanilla Dairy Milk Alternative (page 173)

Soy Velvet Whipped Cream* (page 170) (optional)

TO PREPARE THE PUDDING: Thoroughly grease an 8 by 11 by 2-inch glass baking dish. Scatter half of the bread cubes evenly over the bottom of the dish. Distribute the pears in a single layer on top of the bread.

Sprinkle half of the chocolate and half of the brown sugar evenly over the pears. Scatter the remaining bread and chocolate evenly over the top.

Whisk together the eggs and milk in a large bowl until well blended. Slowly pour the egg mixture over the top of the bread. Set the dish aside for about 20 minutes, periodically pushing the bread down lightly with the back of a fork, until the bread has absorbed much of the egg mixture. Sprinkle the remaining brown sugar on top of the bread. While the bread is soaking, preheat the oven to 325°F.

TO BAKE THE PUDDING: Set the baking dish in a larger pan; transfer to the oven and add enough hot water to the larger pan to reach halfway up the sides of the baking dish. Bake, uncovered, for 1½ hours. The pudding should be slightly soft in the center and crisp on top. Remove from the oven and allow the pudding to cool for 15 minutes before serving. Serve warm with Soy Velvet Whipped Cream.

summer berry pudding

Free of SOY* NUT OIL

SERVES 6

This recipe was inspired by our trip to London, where my husband was served the most beautiful summer pudding. When we returned home, I was determined to create a gluten-free version.

8¹/₂ cups raspberries (reserve ¹/₂ cup for garnish)

1 cup sugar, more or less to taste

3 cups blackberries or marionberries

3 cups blueberries or black currants

1 loaf Fiber-Rich Sandwich Bread (page 137)

Soy Velvet Whipped Cream* (page 170) (optional)

Mint sprigs, for garnish

TO PREPARE THE BREAD: Cut the crust off the bread and slice the loaf into ¹/₂-inch-thick slices. Cut a circle out of 1 slice of the bread to fit in the bottom of a 2-quart glass or ceramic bowl. Line the bottom and sides of the bowl with the remaining bread slices, arranging the slices close together without overlapping, cutting and shaping as needed to cover any gaps.

TO PREPARE THE BERRIES: Combine 8 cups of raspberries and ²/₃ cup of the sugar in a saucepan, stirring to combine. In a separate saucepan, combine 2¹/₂ cups of the blackberries, 2¹/₂ cups of the blueberries, and the remaining ¹/₄ cup of sugar, stirring to combine. Over medium-high heat, bring both mixtures to a boil, stirring occasionally, and cook for 3 to 4 minutes, or until the berries just begin to burst and release their juices; do not overcook. Remove from the heat.

Spoon a layer of raspberries into the bottom of the bowl, followed by the blackberry mixture, alternating layers with the remaining berries. Reserve ¹/₂ cup of the raspberry juice, cover, and refrigerate. Cover the top with the remaining bread slices and press down so that the bread absorbs the juices; cover loosely with a piece of plastic wrap. Set a plate, with a slightly smaller diameter than the bowl, on top of the berries and bread and weight it with heavy cans to compress the layers. Refrigerate overnight.

Remove the pudding from the refrigerator. Remove the cans and plate and allow the pudding to rest about 15 minutes. Using a flexible spatula, loosen the bread from around the bowl. Place a serving platter on top of the bowl, holding it in place, and invert the bowl onto the platter. The bread should be a deep red color all over. Pour the reserved raspberry juice over the pudding taking care to cover any light spots. Garnish with reserved berries, Soy Velvet Whipped Cream, and mint sprigs.

flourless chocolate almond cake

Free of SOY* OIL

MAKES ONE 9-INCH CAKE

Don't let the lengthy instructions dissuade you from making this cake. It's actually easier than it looks and is sure to satisfy an intense chocolate craving. Commercially prepared almond paste often contains wheat; for this reason I have included a recipe for almond paste, which should be made well in advance of the cake. This cake keeps exceptionally well, if covered and refrigerated.

CAKE

8 ounces semisweet dairy-free chocolate*, chopped

³/₄ cup canned light coconut milk

2 teaspoons gluten-free vanilla extract

¹/₄ cup almond meal flour

6 large eggs

¹/₂ cup sugar

GLAZE

²/₃ cup canned light coconut milk

8 ounces bittersweet or semisweet dairy-free chocolate*, finely chopped

1¹/₄ cups sliced almonds, toasted (see page 186)

Almond Paste (page 156)

TO PREPARE THE CAKE: Preheat the oven to 400°F. Line the bottom of a 9-inch springform pan with parchment paper, generously grease the paper and sides of the pan, and set aside.

In a food processor, grind the chocolate into a coarse meal. Heat the coconut milk in a saucepan over medium-high heat, until it just reaches a boil. Pour the milk over the chocolate in the food processor and pulse until smooth. Transfer the chocolate to a large bowl. Stir in the vanilla and almond meal flour.

Using an electric mixer, beat the eggs and sugar on high speed for 4 minutes, or until the mixture has doubled in volume. Fold the eggs into the chocolate mixture until just incorporated. Pour the batter into the prepared pan and bake until a dry crust forms on top but the center is still slightly soft, 20 to 22 minutes. Transfer the pan to a wire rack and allow the cake to cool completely, about 1¹/₂ hours. Refrigerate for 2 hours or overnight to set. The cake will fall as it cools. Before removing the cake from the pan, lightly press down on the top of the cake to compact it further and to even out the crusty top. Remove the sides of the pan. Using the cake pan as a guide, cut out a 9-inch cardboard round and

continued

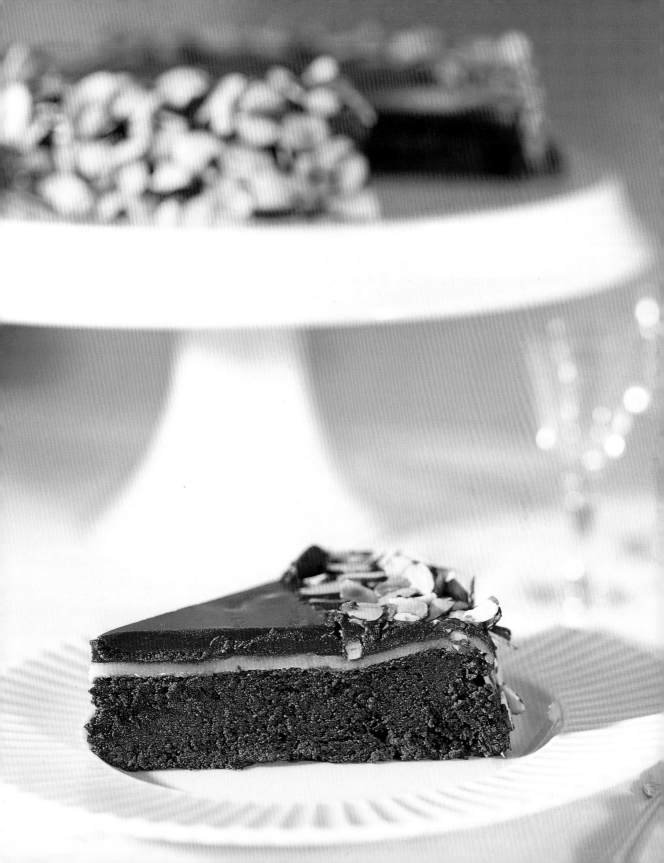

place it on top of the cake. Invert the cake onto the round, gently brush away any large crumbs. The cake can be prepared 1 day ahead if tightly covered and kept at room temperature.

TO FINISH THE CAKE: Roll the almond paste between 2 sheets of plastic wrap to a thickness of about ⅛ inch. Cut out a 9-inch circle, using the bottom of the cake pan as a guide. Place the almond circle atop the cake. Transfer the cake to a wire rack and place the rack over an extra-large bowl. The bowl will be used to catch the excess chocolate glaze.

TO PREPARE THE GLAZE AND DECORATE THE CAKE: Set a small saucepan over low heat and melt the coconut milk and chocolate, stirring until smooth. Remove from the heat and cool until the glaze is almost set but still spreadable. Spread the sides of the cake with just enough glaze to even out any imperfections, taking care not to let any crumbs get into the remaining glaze. Slowly reheat the glaze over low heat until it is smooth and just pourable, but not thin and runny. Pour the remaining glaze into the center of the cake and, working quickly, spread it over the top of the cake and around the sides, working the glaze as little as possible. Allow the glaze to cool slightly. Sprinkle the almonds around the outer edge of the top of the cake, forming a 1½-inch border. Gently press the almonds onto the sides of the cake so they adhere to the glaze. Transfer the cake to a platter and allow the glaze to set for about 30 minutes. Serve at room temperature.

almond paste

1½ cups almond meal flour

¾ cup sugar

3 tablespoons water

1½ tablespoons freshly squeezed lemon juice

TO PREPARE THE ALMOND PASTE: Place the almond meal flour in a food processor. In a medium saucepan combine the sugar, water, and lemon juice over medium-high heat. Stir the mixture until the sugar dissolves and begins to boil. When it begins to boil, start a timer and boil the syrup for 3½ minutes, until it reaches the soft ball stage or until a candy thermometer reaches 240°F. (The soft ball stage is the point at which a drop of boiling syrup dropped in cold water forms a soft ball.) With the motor running, begin pouring the syrup into the processor in a slow stream, and process until fully incorporated, about 2 minutes. Spread a piece of plastic wrap on the counter and spoon the paste onto the center. Shape the paste into a log and wrap tightly in plastic wrap. Refrigerate for 1 week to cure or up to a month. To work with the paste, bring it to room temperature before rolling it out.

tropical fruit crumble

Free of EGG SOY SUGAR OIL

SERVES 6

This is one of my favorite deserts to prepare when time is short and I want to serve something that is sweet yet healthy. Pineapple, mango, dates, and oats are fiber powerhouses and loaded with vitamins A, C, potassium, and copper. If fresh pineapple or mango is unavailable, frozen fruit may be used; simply thaw and cut it into ¹/₂-inch pieces.

FILLING

¹/₄ cup Date Syrup (page 189) or honey

1 teaspoon gluten-free vanilla extract

2¹/₂ cups chopped fresh pineapple, cut into ¹/₂-inch pieces (about half of 1 large pineapple)

2¹/₂ cups chopped ripe mangos, peeled, pitted, and cut into ¹/₂-inch pieces (about 3 mangos)

CRUST

2¹/₂ cups gluten-free rolled oats

¹/₄ cup unsweetened shredded or flaked coconut

1 tablespoon Gluten-Free Flour Mix (page 172)

²/₃ cup Date Syrup (page 189), or ¹/₂ cup honey

Preheat the oven to 350°F. Lightly oil an 8 by 8-inch cake pan or 9-inch deep-dish pie pan with coconut oil and set aside.

TO PREPARE THE FILLING: In a bowl combine the date syrup and vanilla, stirring to blend. Add the pineapple and mango, stirring to incorporate. Set aside.

TO PREPARE THE CRUST AND ASSEMBLE THE DISH: In another bowl combine the oats, coconut, and flour, stirring to blend. Add the date syrup, stirring to fully combine. Transfer two-thirds of the oat mixture to the prepared pan, using a spatula to press the oat mixture into the bottom of the pan and compact it. Pour the fruit mixture over the oats and gently press down with a spatula to compact the fruit. Evenly distribute the remaining oat mixture on top of the fruit to form a crust. Bake the dish 20 to 25 minutes, or until the oats are golden brown. Serve warm.

lemon blueberry tart

Free of EGG SOY* OIL

MAKES ONE 9-INCH TART

Tart yet sweet—a favorite flavor combination that makes this dessert ideal after any meal. The blueberries remain uncooked, keeping them fresh, juicy, and tart.

TART SHELL

1¹/₂ cups almond meal flour

¹/₂ cup Gluten-Free Flour Mix (page 172)

¹/₂ teaspoon xanthan gum

¹/₄ teaspoon salt

1 cup Orange Date Syrup (page 189)

1 tablespoon ice water

¹/₃ cup apricot all-fruit preserves

FILLING

1 (6-ounce) container dairy-free vanilla yogurt*

1 tablespoon freshly squeezed lemon juice

1 tablespoon chopped lemon zest (2 to 3 lemons)

1 teaspoon guar gum

2 cups fresh blueberries, sorted, rinsed, and patted dry with paper towels

Position the rack in the middle of the oven. Preheat the oven to 400°F. Spray a 9-inch tart pan with a removable bottom with cooking spray and line the bottom of the pan with parchment paper. Set aside.

TO PREPARE THE TART SHELL: Combine the almond meal flour, flour, xanthan gum, and salt in a bowl and whisk together until well blended. Add the date syrup and water, and mix quickly with your hands until the dough holds together to form a ball.

Form the dough into a slightly flattened disk and place between 2 sheets of plastic wrap. Using a rolling pin, roll out the dough into an 11- to 12-inch round, periodically lifting and repositioning the plastic wrap over the dough. Remove the top layer of plastic wrap and invert the dough into the prepared pan. Gently press the dough into the pan, removing any excess. Weight with dried beans or pie weights. Bake until the sides are set, about 15 minutes. Remove the foil and weights. Bake until the shell is a deep golden brown, about 15 minutes longer. Transfer to a wire rack and cool completely.

Heat the preserves in a small saucepan until melted. With a pastry brush, use 2 tablespoons of the glaze to coat the tart shell and set aside, about 1 hour, reserving the remaining preserves. Cover the shell and keep at room temperature. It can be made 1 day ahead.

TO PREPARE THE FILLING: Combine the yogurt, lemon juice, zest, and guar gum in a bowl. Whisk until well blended and the yogurt begins to thicken, about 2 minutes.

TO ASSEMBLE THE TART: Spoon the yogurt mixture into the tart shell and smooth it with a rubber spatula. Gently arrange the fruit on top of the filling, distributing evenly. Rewarm the apricot glaze over low heat, until just warm, and brush over the berries. Refrigerate for at least 1 hour, or overnight, before serving.

spiced apple tart

Free of EGG SOY OIL

MAKES ONE 9-INCH TART

This simply delicious and easy-to-assemble tart is a seasonal family favorite. Although this version is made with apples, pears would work equally as well, or for a burst of summer flavor, pitted, halved apricots pair beautifully with the almond crust.

Tart shell (see page 158)

FILLING

2 pounds pippin, Golden Delicious, or McIntosh apples (about 4 medium)

2 tablespoons sugar

1 teaspoon ground cinnamon

Prepare the tart shell (page 158), but do not pre-bake or glaze with apricot preserves.

TO PREPARE THE FILLING: In a bowl combine the sugar and cinnamon, stirring to blend. Peel, quarter, and core the apples, then slice them into $1/8$- to $1/4$-inch-thick slices. Transfer the apple slices to the sugar mixture and toss to coat. Arrange the first row of apple slices around the outer edge of the tart shell, forming a circle. Make the next row by placing the apples closely against the first. Continue the process until you reach the center. Cover the edge of the crust with a ring of aluminum foil to prevent burning, taking care not to cover the apples.

Bake the tart for 45 minutes. Remove the foiled edge and bake 15 minutes longer. Serve warm or at room temperature. The tart can be made 1 day ahead. Cool completely, cover, and keep at room temperature.

currant apple brandy rice cake

MAKES ONE 9-INCH CAKE

This soft, moist rice cake, reminiscent of rice pudding, is deeply satisfying; with just a hint of brandy, the gentle sweetness of apples and currants makes for comfort food at its best.

1/2 cup brandy

1/3 cup dried currants or raisins

1 large Granny Smith apple, peeled, cored, and diced

1 1/2 cups short-grain brown rice (such as arborio)

5 cups Dairy Milk Alternative (page 173)

1 1/4 cups sugar

1/4 teaspoon ground cinnamon

4 large eggs, separated

1 teaspoon gluten-free vanilla extract

Soy Velvet Whipped Cream* (page 170) (optional)

TO MAKE THE CAKE: Warm the brandy in a small saucepan over low heat and stir in the currants and apple. Remove the pan from the heat and set aside.

Combine the rice, milk, 1/4 cup of the sugar, and cinnamon in a large saucepan over medium-high heat. Bring the mixture just to a boil, decrease the heat to low, cover, and simmer, stirring occasionally, until the liquid is absorbed, about 1 hour.

Line the bottom of a 9-inch springform pan with parchment paper. Reserve 1 tablespoon of the sugar, and place the remaining sugar in a small skillet over medium-high heat. Cook the sugar, without stirring, until it begins to melt, about 2 minutes. Continue cooking, stirring constantly, until the sugar is melted and golden, about 3 minutes. Working quickly, pour the melted sugar (caramel) into the prepared pan and tilt to coat the bottom and the sides. Set aside to cool.

Preheat the oven to 375°F. Strain the currants and apples, using a fine sieve, and discard the brandy. Stir the egg yolks, currants, apple, and vanilla into the rice mixture until blended. Beat the egg whites in a seperate bowl until foamy. Add the reserved 1 tablespoon of sugar and continue to beat until soft peaks form. Fold the egg whites into the rice until incorporated. Pour the mixture into the caramelized pan, and set the pan in a larger pan partially filled with water, halfway up the inner pan. Bake, uncovered, until golden brown and a knife inserted in the center comes out clean, about 1 hour. Transfer the cake to a rack and cool to room temperature, about 1 hour. Remove the sides of the pan and place a large platter on the top of the cake. Invert the cake onto the platter and remove the parchment paper. Serve each slice with a dollop of Soy Velvet Whipped Cream.

german apple soufflé à la mode

Free of SOY NUT* OIL

SERVES 4

This pancake-like soufflé is surprisingly easy to make but looks impressive. Be sure to have your guests gathered at the table, because when the soufflé is pulled from the oven it quickly deflates. Serve it topped with a scoop of Coconut Ice Cream (page 163).

APPLES

1 pound pippin or Granny Smith apples, peeled, cored, and thinly sliced

2 tablespoons sugar

1 tablespoon freshly squeezed lemon juice

1 tablespoon brandy (optional)

½ teaspoon ground cinnamon

BATTER

3 large eggs

¾ cup Dairy Milk Alternative (page 173)

¾ cup Gluten-Free Flour Mix (page 172)

¼ teaspoon salt

TOPPINGS

Pure maple syrup, warmed

Coconut Ice Cream* (page 163)

TO PREPARE THE APPLES: Combine the apples, sugar, lemon juice, brandy, and cinnamon in a bowl and toss to coat the apples. Heat a large sauté pan over medium-high heat. Add the apple mixture and sauté the apples until just softened, 6 to 8 minutes. Meanwhile, preheat the oven to 450°F. Spray an 8 by 11 by 2-inch baking dish with cooking spray. Distribute the apples evenly over the bottom of the dish.

TO PREPARE THE BATTER: Whisk together the eggs and milk in a bowl until well blended. Add the flour and salt and stir until just combined. The batter will be slightly lumpy. Slowly pour the batter over the apples. Bake until the soufflé is golden brown and puffed, 20 to 22 minutes. Cut into wedges and serve immediately on individual dessert plates, with a scoop of Coconut Ice Cream (page 163) and a drizzle of maple syrup.

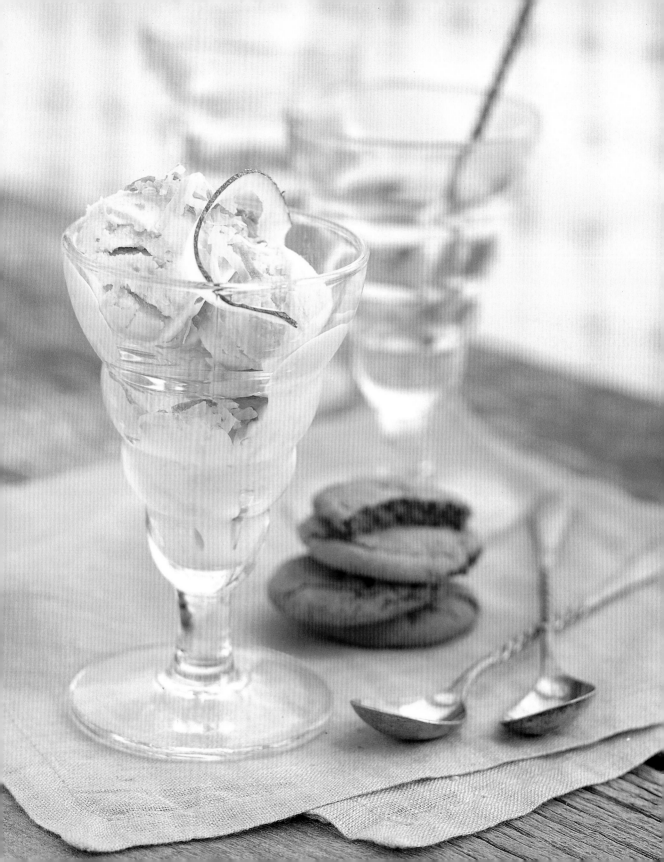

coconut ice cream

Free of EGG SOY

MAKES 1 QUART

This ice cream is so decadently rich, you'll find that a little goes a long way. Use this versatile recipe as a base and customize it with any of the variations below or let your imagination run wild and create your own flavor. Serve this ice cream slightly softened, straight form the ice cream maker.

Note: This recipe calls for an ice cream maker. Read manufacturer's instructions before starting the recipe in case of any advanced preparation.

1 (13.5 ounce) can unsweetened coconut milk

2 cups coconut milk beverage

$3/4$ cup sugar

1 teaspoon guar gum

$1/8$ teaspoon salt

Combine the coconut milk, coconut beverage, sugar, guar gum, and salt in a blender, cover, and whirl at top speed until thoroughly blended, about 2 minutes. Place the blender jar in the refrigerator and chill for 1 hour. Remove from the refrigerator and pulse the mixture to incorporate. Pour the mixture into an ice cream maker and process according to the manufacturer's directions.

TO STORE THE ICE CREAM: Transfer it to a plastic container with a tight-fitting lid. Place a piece of plastic wrap on top of the ice cream, cover, and freeze. To serve, allow the ice cream to soften slightly at room temperature.

VARIATIONS: TOASTED COCONUT ICE CREAM

Preheat the oven to 325°F. Position a rack in the middle of the oven. Spread $1/8$ cup flaked coconut in a thin layer on a small rimmed baking sheet and toast it in the oven, stirring frequently, until lightly golden, about 4 minutes. Set aside to cool. Stir the cooled flakes into the ice cream mixture and process as instructed.

CHOCOLATE CHUNK COCONUT ICE CREAM

Add 4 ounces of semisweet dairy-free dark chocolate, coarsely chopped, and process as instructed.

REDUCED SUGAR COCONUT ICE CREAM

Reduce the sugar to $1/4$ cup and add $1/4$ to $1/2$ teaspoon pure stevia extract powder or $1/2$ to 1 teaspoon of liquid stevia extract, tasting and adding in small increments as needed. Process as instructed.

pumpkin cheesecake

Free of `OIL`

MAKES ONE 9-INCH CAKE

This cheesecake is so rich, creamy, and flavorful, it's hard to believe it is dairy-free and gluten-free. Making it a day ahead allows the cake to settle, giving it the dense texture of a dairy cheesecake, but without all the fat.

¼ cup Spicy Ginger Cookie crumbs (page 166) or gluten-free graham cracker crumbs

32 ounces firm silken tofu, drained

1½ cups sugar

5 large eggs

⅓ cup Gluten-Free Flour Mix (page 172)

¼ teaspoon salt

1 (15-ounce) can solid-pack pumpkin puree

5 teaspoons pumpkin pie spice

Soy Velvet Whipped Cream* (page 170), for garnish (optional)

Preheat the oven to 325°F.

TO PREPARE THE PAN AND THE CRUST: Using dairy-free margarine, thoroughly coat the bottom and sides of a 9-inch springform pan. Place the Spicy Ginger Cookie crumbs in the pan and shake to coat the bottom and sides of the pan, leaving the excess in the bottom; set aside.

TO PREPARE AND BAKE THE CHEESECAKE: In a food processor, pulse the tofu until creamy. Gradually add the sugar. Add the eggs, 1 at a time, pulsing well after each addition. Add the flour, salt, pumpkin, and pumpkin pie spice. Pour the mixture into the prepared pan.

TO BAKE AND SERVE THE PIE: Bake until firm, about 1½ hours. Turn off the heat. The top of the cake will have cracked during baking. Open the oven door slightly and let the cake cool for 30 minutes in the oven. Cool completely on a wire rack, about 2 hours. Remove the sides of the pan, cover, and refrigerate. Before serving, allow the cheesecake to return to room temperature. Garnish each slice with Soy Velvet Whipped Cream.

rum caramel flan

Free of SOY NUT OIL

SERVES 6

For Valentine's Day. I like to bake this flan in heart-shaped ramekins and serve them on white plates garnished with fresh raspberries.

CARAMEL

²⁄₃ **cup sugar**

5 tablespoons water

1 tablespoon dark rum

CUSTARD

2 cups Dairy Milk Alternative (page 173)

1 teaspoon arrowroot or cornstarch

¹⁄₄ **cup sugar**

4 large egg yolks

2 large eggs

¹⁄₂ **teaspoon gluten-free vanilla extract**

1 tablespoon dark rum

TO MAKE THE CARAMEL: Arrange six ³⁄₄-cup ramekins or custard cups in a 13 by 9 by 2-inch baking dish. Combine the sugar and water in a small sauté pan over medium-high heat and cook, stirring constantly, until the sugar has dissolved and the syrup turns a golden color, 2 to 3 minutes. Add the rum, stir, and cook for about 30 seconds.

Remove from the heat and immediately pour the syrup into the ramekins, dividing it equally. If the syrup begins to harden before you have finished, return the pan to the heat and stir until it liquefies.

TO PREPARE THE CUSTARD: Preheat the oven to 350°F. Combine the milk, arrowroot, and sugar in a heavy medium saucepan. Stir over medium-low heat, until the mixture is warm and the sugar has dissolved, 2 to 3 minutes. Remove from the heat. Whisk the egg yolks and eggs in a medium bowl to blend. Gradually whisk in the warm milk, vanilla, and rum. Divide the mixture equally among the ramekins. Pour enough hot water into the baking dish to come halfway up the sides of the ramekins, being careful not to get any water in the custard mixture. Cover the dish with aluminum foil and bake the custards until the center moves slightly when gently shaken, about 35 minutes. Remove from the pan and place ramekins on a wire rack to cool for about 1 hour. Cover each with plastic wrap and chill at least 4 hours or overnight.

To serve, loosen the sides of each flan by running a thin, sharp knife around the edge. Cover the cup with a rimmed dessert plate and, holding both together, quickly invert. Remove the ramekin and serve.

spicy ginger cookies

MAKES 18 COOKIES

These delectable cookies are surprisingly moist and rich, contain minimal oil, no refined sugar, and have a zippy ginger zing. Try eating them warm from the oven with an icy cold glass of your favorite dairy-free milk. They're also wonderful chopped up and sprinkled over a baked apple or poached pears, and serves as a delicious crust for the Pumpkin Cheesecake (page 164).

2^1/$_2$ cups Gluten-Free Flour Mix (page 172)

2 teaspoons baking soda

1 tablespoon ground ginger

1 teaspoon ground cinnamon

^{1}/$_4$ teaspoon ground nutmeg

^{1}/$_8$ teaspoon ground cloves

4 tablespoons crystallized ginger, finely chopped

^{3}/$_4$ cup Date Syrup (page 189)

3 tablespoons water

1 tablespoon canola oil* (optional)

6 prunes, pitted

1 large egg

^{1}/$_4$ cup blackstrap molasses

TO MAKE THE DOUGH: Combine the flour, baking soda, ginger, cinnamon, nutmeg, and cloves in a bowl. Mix together with a whisk until well blended. Add the ginger and stir to combine. Set aside.

In a blender, combine the date syrup, water, oil, prunes, egg, and molasses. Cover and whirl at top speed, scraping down the sides of the container as needed, until the mixture is smooth, about 2 minutes. Pour the wet ingredients into the dry ingredients and, using a rubber spatula, stir well to combine. Cover the bowl with plastic wrap and allow the dough to rest for 15 minutes. Meanwhile, preheat the oven to 350°F and line an insulated baking sheet with parchment paper.

TO SHAPE AND BAKE THE COOKIES: Spoon the dough by the tablespoonful, 2 inches apart, onto the prepared baking sheet. Repeat with the remaining dough, using your fingers, shape and smooth the cookies, flattening them slightly. Bake for 10 minutes. Watch the cookies carefully; over-baking them will make them dry and hard. Transfer the cookies to a wire rack to cool.

TO STORE THE COOKIES: Place the fully cooled cookies in an airtight container for up to 3 days or freeze for longer storage.

almond biscotti

Free of SOY OIL

MAKES 14 BISCOTTI

Biscotti are classic Italian twice-baked cookies, and what most consider the ultimate dunking cookies for hot coffee. The first time I encountered biscotti, I was twenty years old with a backpack on my back, traipsing around the Tuscan countryside. I remember resting at a streetside café and watching people dunk something in their coffee. I ordered the same and fell in love at first bite.

1¹/₂ cups Gluten-Free Flour Mix (page 172)

1 cup almond meal flour

1 teaspoon gluten-free baking powder

¹/₄ teaspoon baking soda

¹/₈ teaspoon nutmeg

¹/₂ cup sliced almonds, toasted (see page 186)

³/₄ cup sugar

2 large eggs

1 teaspoon almond extract

Position a rack in the center of the oven and preheat the oven to 300°F.

TO PREPARE THE DOUGH: Combine the flour, almond meal flour, baking powder, baking soda, and nutmeg in a bowl and mix together with a whisk until well blended. Add the almonds and stir to incorporate. Using an electric mixer on medium speed, beat the sugar, eggs, and almond extract in a large bowl until smooth, about 2 minutes. Using a large spoon, stir the flour mixture into the sugar mixture until just combined; the dough will be sticky. Turn the dough out onto a flat, nonstick surface and with your hands, shape the dough into a log approximately 10 inches long by 3¹/₂ inches wide by 1 inch thick.

TO BAKE THE BISCOTTI: Line an insulated baking sheet with parchment paper. Transfer the log to the prepared baking sheet. Reshape if needed. Bake the log until it is dry and slightly firm to the touch, about 40 minutes, or until light golden brown. Transfer the log to a wire rack and cool for 10 minutes.

Carefully transfer the log to a cutting board. With a serrated knife and using a sawing motion, cut the log into ³/₄-inch-thick slices. Stand the slices upright on the parchment-lined baking sheet and bake 30 minutes. Remove the biscotti from the oven and transfer to a wire rack to cool completely, about 1¹/₂ hours. The biscotti will continue to harden as they cool.

TO STORE THE COOKIES: Place the fully cooled cookies in an airtight container. They will keep for up to 1 week.

bird's nest cookies

Free of EGG SOY SUGAR OIL

MAKES 18 TO 24 COOKIES

As cookies go, it's hard to get healthier than these little gems—they're vegan with no refined oil or sugar. I grew up calling these tasty little wonders "bird's nests," yet many others know them as thumbprint cookies. Fill them with your favorite preserves or with an assortment of preserves. Either way, they make colorful gift cookies or a pretty addition to a cookie platter.

$3/4$ cup **Gluten-Free Flour Mix (page 172)**

$3/4$ cup **almond meal flour**

$1/2$ cup **gluten-free quick oats**

1 teaspoon **gluten-free baking powder**

$1/2$ teaspoon **xanthan gum**

$1/2$ teaspoon **ground cinnamon**

$1/4$ teaspoon **salt**

$1/2$ cup **Orange Date Syrup (page 189)**

$1/3$ cup **smooth almond butter**

1 teaspoon **gluten-free vanilla extract**

$1/4$ cup **all-fruit preserves**

Preheat the oven to 350°F. Line an insulated baking sheet with parchment paper.

TO PREPARE THE DOUGH: In a large bowl, whisk together the date syrup, almond butter, and vanilla. In a separate bowl, combine the flour, almond meal, oats, baking powder, xanthan gum, cinnamon, and salt, and mix together with a wire whisk until well blended. Add the dry ingredients to the wet ingredients and stir until incorporated.

TO SHAPE AND BAKE THE COOKIES: Spoon about 1 tablespoon of the dough into the palm of your hand and roll it into a round ball about $1^1/_2$-inches in diameter. Transfer the balls, about 1 inch apart, to the prepared baking sheet. Gently press your thumb in the center of each ball, creating a well, and gently reshape the cookie as needed. Spoon $1/2$ teaspoon preserves in the hollow of each cookie. Bake until set, 12 to 14 minutes. Remove the cookies from the oven and, using a wide spatula, transfer the cookies to a wire rack to cool completely.

TO STORE THE COOKIES: Place the fully cooled cookies in an airtight container for up to 1 week, separating them with a layer of plastic wrap, or freeze for longer storage.

cake brownies *with* orange essence

Free of   EGG   SOY*   NUT   SUGAR   OIL

MAKES 20 BROWNIES

Not your traditional dense brownie loaded with fat and sugar, this version has just the right balance of chocolate and orange to dazzle the taste buds. This recipe is fiber rich, free of added fat and processed sugar, and is about as healthy as a sweet treat can get.

2 cups Gluten-Free Flour Mix (page 172)

1¼ cups unsweetened cocoa powder

1 tablespoon ground flax meal

2 teaspoons baking soda

½ teaspoon xanthan gum

1½ tablespoons orange zest (about 1 orange)

1 cup orange Date Syrup (page 189)

1 cup Dairy Milk Alternative (page 174)

½ cup plain dairy-free yogurt*

8 prunes, pitted

1 teaspoon gluten-free vanilla extract

Preheat the oven to 425°F. Spray an 8 by 8-inch baking pan with cooking spray and line the bottom and sides with parchment paper. Set aside.

TO PREPARE THE BROWNIES: Combine the flour, cocoa, flax, baking soda, and xanthan gum in a bowl and mix together with a wire whisk until blended. Add the zest and mix to blend. Set aside.

Combine the date syrup, milk, yogurt, prunes, and vanilla in a blender. Cover and whirl at top speed, scraping down the sides as needed, until the mixture is smooth, about 2 minutes. Pour the wet ingredients into the dry ingredients and, using a rubber spatula, stir well to combine. Pour the batter into the prepared pan, smoothing out the top, and bake until the brownies spring back when touched, 20 to 25 minutes. Cool the brownies completely before cutting into squares.

chocolate orange pudding

Free of EGG NUT OIL

SERVES 4

Sometimes, all I want for dessert without being too "bad" is some chocolate pudding. In this version, I've combined three of my favorite flavors, chocolate, orange, and ginger, for a luscious and creamy treat.

1 (12-ounce) package firm silken tofu, drained

$1/3$ cup unsweetened cocoa powder

2 tablespoons pure maple syrup

2 tablespoons Orange Date Syrup (page 189)

1 teaspoon gluten-free vanilla extract

Soy Velvet Whipped Cream or other dairy-free whipped cream

1 tablespoon chopped crystallized ginger, for garnish

2 teaspoons orange zest, for garnish

Combine the tofu, cocoa powder, maple syrup, date syrup, and vanilla in a blender. Cover and puree the mixture, scraping down the sides as needed, until the pudding is smooth and creamy, about 2 minutes. Transfer the pudding to individual serving bowls, cover, and refrigerate for at least 1 hour. Top with a dollop of whipped cream, and sprinkle with crystallized ginger and zest.

soy velvet whipped cream

MAKES 2 CUPS

1 (12-ounce) package firm silken tofu, drained

2 tablespoons Date Syrup (page 189)

2 tablespoons pure maple syrup

1 teaspoon gluten-free vanilla extract

$1/4$ teaspoon guar gum ($1/4$ teaspoon more for a firmer cream)

Place all the ingredients in a blender, cover, and whirl at top speed, scraping down the sides often, until smooth, about 2 minutes. Transfer to a container with a tight-fitting lid and refrigerate for 1 hour or for up to 3 days. Stir to blend before using.

basics

The basic recipes in this chapter are the backbone of many of the recipes included in this book, from the gluten-free flour mix, to making your own fresh dairy milk alternative, yogurt, and cheese, to flavorful stocks and sauces, to tips on cooking legumes and grains. All of the recipes here are surprisingly uncomplicated to prepare and add superior flavor to any dish.

gluten-free flour mix

Free of EGG SOY NUT SUGAR OIL

MAKES 3 CUPS

Use this recipe as an excellent all-purpose, gluten-free substitute anytime a recipe calls for flour. It can easily be doubled or tripled ensuring that you always have gluten-free flour on hand.

1¼ cups brown or white rice flour

¾ cup potato starch (do not use potato flour)

½ cup tapioca flour or arrowroot flour

½ cup sorghum flour or garbanzo bean flour

Combine the rice flour, potato starch, tapioca flour, and sorghum flour in a large bowl. Mix together with a whisk until thoroughly combined. Transfer the flour mixture to an airtight container and refrigerate until ready to use. This gluten-free flour mix will keep for 4 months in the refrigerator.

NOTE: This flour mix does not contain either xantham or guar gum. For more information, see page 17.

dairy milk alternative

MAKES 3 CUPS

All of the recipes in this book have been developed to interchangeably use commercially available almond milk, soy milk, rice milk, hemp milk, or coconut beverage. However, the satisfaction of preparing your own fresh dairy-free nut milk is both simple and delicious. I am partial to raw almonds and cashews, but this recipe is perfectly suitable for any of your favorite nuts. Start by selecting organic, raw nuts—choose from almonds, cashews, hazelnuts, Brazil nuts, pine nuts, or macadamia nuts. This unsweetened nut milk can be used in any of the recipes in this book. If a recipe calls for a vanilla version or you prefer a slightly sweetened milk, add in the optional ingredients.

1 cup raw almonds, soaked for 10 to 12 hours in cold water

4 cups cold filtered water

1 tablespoon Date Syrup (page 189), brown rice syrup, or maple syrup (optional)

$^1/_2$ teaspoon gluten-free vanilla extract, to taste

Using a colander, drain the soaked almonds and rinse under cold running water. In a blender, combine the almonds, water, and optional ingredients, if desired. Cover the blender and whirl the mixture at top speed until creamy, about 1 minute. Line a fine-mesh sieve with a double layer of cheesecloth and place it over a large bowl. Pour the almond mixture into the strainer and allow it to fully drain, about 5 minutes. Gather up the corners of the cheesecloth and squeeze the mixture to extract any remaining liquid. Reserve the pulp for another use (see Edamame Nut Pâté, page 127). Transfer the milk to a glass container with a tight-fitting lid, cover, and refrigerate for up to 3 days.

nut milk yogurt

Free of EGG SOY SUGAR OIL

MAKES 4 CUPS

Although commercially available dairy-free yogurt made from soy, almond, coconut milk, and rice milk are good substitutes for dairy yogurt, nothing compares to making your own; it allows you to customize the yogurt to accommodate your food intolerance and your taste. It's essential to use fresh nut milk (see page 173) because store-bought milks contain additives that make it difficult to achieve success. Homemade yogurt is thinner than commercial brands, so adding a thickener, such as guar gum, agar agar, arrowroot, or dairy-free milk powder are all good options. For this recipe you'll need an instant-read thermometer and either a yogurt maker (preferred) or heating pad. If using a heating pad, it will need to be one that stays on, not the automatic shut-off type. Please note that not all yogurt starters are dairy-free, so be sure to check the packaging. You'll find online dairy-free manufacturers and distributors section in the resources (page 192).

4 cups unsweetened Dairy Milk Alternative (page 173)

3 tablespoons Date Syrup (page 189)

$^1/_2$ teaspoon guar gum (optional)

$^1/_4$ teaspoon gluten-free vanilla extract (optional)

$^1/_4$ to $^1/_2$ teaspoon dairy-free yogurt starter

TO STERILIZE THE JARS: In a large pot fitted with a rack or steamer insert, place 4 upright 8-ounce glass canning jars on the rack. Fill the pot with enough water to cover the tops of the jars and bring to a boil. Boil the jars for 10 minutes to sterilize. Using tongs, carefully lift the jars out of the pot and invert the jars on a cooling rack to cool.

TO PREPARE THE YOGURT: Meanwhile, in a saucepan over medium heat, add the milk, date syrup, and guar gum, stirring to blend. Heat the mixture to 180°F, stirring frequently; do not allow the mixture to boil. Turn off the heat, stir in the vanilla and let the milk cool to 105° to 110°F. (This cooling step is very important; if the milk is too hot it will kill the live probiotic yogurt starter.) Once the milk has cooled add the yogurt starter and whisk until fully incorporated. Pour the mixture into the yogurt maker and incubate according to the manufacturer's directions. If you do not have a yogurt maker, place a heating pad on the kitchen counter and set it to medium. Divide the milk mixture equally among the sterilized jars. Arrange the uncapped jars on the heating pad and cover with a double layer bath towel. Incubate the yogurt at 115°F to 120°F for 9 to 12 hours. The longer it rests, the firmer and tangier the yogurt will become. Screw on the lids and refrigerate for 4 hours to stop the acid development. The yogurt will keep for 1 week in the refrigerator. Serve it plain or add your favorite fruit.

creamy macadamia pine nut cheese

Free of EGG SOY SUGAR OIL

MAKES 1¹/₂ CUPS

Most raw nut cheeses require soaking the nuts for several hours or overnight, but when I get a hankering for cheese, I don't want to wait for the nuts to soak or culture. For this recipe I chose two nuts that do not require pre-soaking and will yield creamy, rich-tasting cheese in less than 10 minutes! This simple raw nut cheese makes a nice addition to the Rustic Mushroom Pizza (page 98) or Rustic Heirloom Pesto Pizza (page 96) or can be used as a spread or anytime a creamy cheese or ricotta is called for in a recipe.

- **2 cups raw macadamia nuts (not dry roasted)**
- **¹/₄ cup raw pine nuts**
- **¹/₂ cup filtered water (or ³/₄ cup water for a softer cheese)**
- **1 tablespoon freshly squeezed lemon juice**
- **2 teaspoons apple cider vinegar**
- **¹/₂ teaspoon onion powder**
- **¹/₂ teaspoon sea salt**

Combine the macadamia nuts, pine nuts, water, lemon juice, vinegar, onion powder, and salt in a food processor or high-speed blender. Process the mixture, scraping down the sides of the processor with a rubber spatula as needed, and puree until smooth and creamy, about 4 minutes. Use immediately or store in an airtight glass container in the refrigerator for up to 2 days. For longer storage, divide into portion sizes, wrap in plastic wrap, and freeze for up to 1 week.

chicken stock

Free of EGG SOY NUT SUGAR OIL

MAKES 8 TO 10 CUPS

The next time you roast or grill a chicken, save the bones, wing tips, back, and neck, and store them in a large plastic freezer bag in the freezer. When you have collected 4 pounds' worth, you're ready to make homemade chicken stock.

4 pounds chicken bones, wing tips, backs, and necks

2 carrots, peeled, trimmed, and cut into 2-inch pieces

3 stalks celery with leaves, quartered

1 large onion, quartered

8 sprigs flat-leaf parsley, ends trimmed

3 sprigs thyme

1 bay leaf

3 whole black peppercorns

TO PREPARE THE STOCK: Combine the chicken bones, carrots, celery, and onion in a large stockpot. Add water to cover and bring to a rapid boil over high heat; skim off and discard any foam that rises to the top. Decrease the heat to low and add the parsley, thyme, bay leaf, and peppercorns. Simmer, partially covered, periodically skimming off any residue that rises to the top, until reduced by half, 3 to 4 hours.

Remove the pot from the heat and strain the stock into a large nonmetallic bowl. Allow the stock to cool, uncovered, at room temperature for about 1 hour.

When cool, cover the stock with plastic wrap and transfer to the refrigerator until the fat solidifies and rises to the surface, about 2 hours. Using a large, flat spoon, remove and discard the fat. The stock is now ready for use, or it can be frozen and stored for later.

TO FURTHER CLARIFY THE STOCK: Place the refrigerated stock in a large pot and reheat until the stock has just liquefied and is no longer in a gelatinous state, 2 to 3 minutes. Line a fine-mesh strainer with cheesecloth. Place the strainer over a clean bowl and slowly pour the stock into the strainer, eliminating any sediment and peppercorns.

STORAGE TIPS: Pour the cooled stock into ice cube trays and freeze. When the stock has frozen solid, unmold the trays and transfer the cubes to plastic freezer bags. Freeze until ready to use. The stock will keep, covered, in the refrigerator for up to 3 days, or in the freezer for 2 to 3 months.

vegetable stock

MAKES 7 CUPS

This is a full-bodied stock prepared entirely from fresh vegetables and takes less time to cook than stocks made from meat. It can be substituted for chicken stock when you need to turn a vegetable-based recipe into a vegan one.

4 carrots, peeled, trimmed, and cut into 2-inch pieces

1 leek, dark green part only, chopped

1 large turnip, trimmed and cut into 2-inch pieces

1 large russet potato, peeled and cut into 2-inch pieces

3 stalks celery with leaves, quartered

2 large onions, quartered

2 cloves garlic, unpeeled and crushed

6 sprigs flat-leaf parsley

4 sprigs thyme

2 sprigs oregano or marjoram

2 bay leaves

8 whole black peppercorns

TO PREPARE THE STOCK: Combine the carrots, leek, turnip, potato, celery, onion, and garlic in a large stockpot. Add enough water to cover by 2 inches (about 10 cups). Bring to a rapid boil over high heat. Decrease the heat to low and add the parsley, thyme, oregano, bay leaves, and peppercorns. Simmer, uncovered, for $1\frac{1}{2}$ hours. Line a fine-mesh sieve with cheesecloth. Place the sieve over a clean bowl and slowly pour in the stock, straining out any sediment and peppercorns. With the back of a large spoon, lightly press on the vegetables to extract as much liquid as possible, then discard the vegetables.

STORAGE TIPS: Pour the cooled stock into ice cube trays and freeze. When the stock has frozen solid, unmold the trays and transfer the cubes to plastic freezer bags. Freeze until ready to use. The stock will keep, covered, in the refrigerator for up to 3 days, or in the freezer for 2 to 3 months.

herbed tomato sauce

Free of EGG SOY NUT

MAKES 2 CUPS

Depending on the size of my tomato crop, I often double or triple this recipe, freezing or canning the extra sauce and enjoying it during the winter months. Enliven it with capers, roasted peppers, and anchovy.

2^1/$_2$ **pounds medium-size, vine-ripened tomatoes**

2 tablespoons olive oil (or steam-sauté, see page 18)

1 large yellow onion, minced

3 cloves garlic, minced

1 bay leaf

3 sprigs thyme

1 teaspoon salt

^{1}/$_4$ teaspoon freshly ground black pepper

Sugar, if needed

^{1}/$_4$ cup chopped fresh basil

1 tablespoon minced flat-leaf parsley

TO PREPARE THE TOMATOES: Fill a large, deep bowl with ice water and set aside. Bring a large pot of water to a boil over high heat. Immerse the tomatoes in the boiling water for 10 to 45 seconds or until the tomato skin cracks. Using a large slotted spoon, quickly transfer the tomatoes to the ice bath for about 30 seconds. Lift the tomatoes out, allow them to cool briefly, and then pull off and discard the skin. Cut out the cores, halve the tomatoes horizontally, and squeeze out and discard the juice and seeds. Finely chop the tomatoes.

TO MAKE THE SAUCE: Heat the olive oil in a large saucepan over medium-high heat and sauté the onion until softened and slightly browned, about 5 minutes. Stir in the garlic and sauté for 1 minute. Add the tomatoes, bay leaf, thyme, salt, and pepper. Bring to a boil and decrease the heat to low. Simmer the sauce, uncovered, for 20 to 30 minutes, stirring occasionally. Taste and correct the seasonings. If the sauce is very acidic, add a pinch or more of sugar to taste. The finished sauce will have a slight texture to it. If you prefer a smooth, refined sauce, pass the sauce through a food mill or puree it in a blender. Stir in the basil and parsley. Check the consistency. If you like a thicker sauce, return it to the saucepan and cook it over medium-low heat until the desired consistency is reached. The sauce will thicken as it cools. Transfer the sauce to a nonmetallic container with a tight-fitting lid and refrigerate for up to 5 days.

chopped tomatoes

MAKES 3 CUPS

Used as a base in many recipes, these skinned and chopped tomatoes are a flavorful addition to light sauces, soups, and pastas. If desired, try seasoning the tomatoes lightly with salt and pepper and fresh basil—either whole or finely chopped. These chopped tomatoes freeze beautifully, preserving the taste of summer for enjoyment later in the year.

1¹/₂ **pounds medium-size vine-ripened tomatoes**

Fill a large, deep bowl with ice water and set aside. Bring a large pot of water to a boil over high heat. Immerse the tomatoes in the boiling water until the tomato skins crack, 10 to 45 seconds. Using a large slotted spoon, quickly transfer the tomatoes to the ice bath for about 30 seconds. Lift the tomatoes out, allow them to cool briefly, and then pull off and discard the skin. Cut out the cores, coarsely chop the tomatoes, and place them in a large bowl along with their juices until ready to use, or refrigerate for up to 4 days.

STORAGE TIPS: Freeze 1 cup of chopped tomatoes per resealable plastic freezer bag, so you can easily portion them out in recipes. They'll keep for 6 months in the freezer.

dried beans *and* legumes

Free of   EGG   SOY   NUT   SUGAR   OIL

MAKES 4 CUPS

If time is short, canned beans are a great alternative to dried and are just as nutritious as their dried counterpart. Adding a strip of kombu, a sea vegetable, to your pot of beans will help with their digestibility and boost the mineral content.

1 pound dried beans

6 to 8 cups water

2 strips kombu, about 2 by 4 inches (optional)

TO CLEAN THE BEANS AND PREPARE THEM FOR SOAKING:
Place dried beans on a clean, flat surface, preferably light in color to visually aid in the sorting. Sort through the beans and discard any pebbles or chaff. Place the sorted beans in a colander and rinse with cold running water. Dried beans can take a long time to cook unless they have been soaked prior to cooking. You can shorten their cooking time by using one of the following soaking methods.

QUICK SOAKING METHOD: Combine beans and enough water to cover them in a large stockpot. Bring to a rapid boil over high heat and boil for about 2 minutes. Remove the pot from the heat,

cover tightly, and allow the beans to soak for 1 hour. Drain the soaked beans in a colander and rinse them under warm running water.

OVERNIGHT SOAKING METHOD: Combine the beans and enough water to cover them in a large stockpot. Let the beans soak overnight. Drain the soaked beans in a colander and rinse them under cold running water.

TO COOK THE BEANS: Combine the rinsed soaked beans and enough water to cover them in a large stockpot. Add the kombu. Bring the pot to a rapid boil over high heat, partially cover the pot, and reduce the heat to a gentle, rolling boil. Cook the beans until tender, using the approximate cooking times listed below. Check the beans periodically and add more water if necessary to keep them immersed. Drain the beans and use as needed.

APPROXIMATE COOKING TIMES FOR SOAKED DRIED BEANS	
Bean	**Cooking Time**
Aduki and cannellini	1 to 1½ hours
Anasazi, black (turtle), great Northern, kidney, and pinto	1½ to 2 hours
Garbanzo (chickpeas)	2½ to 3 hours
Lima (large and baby)	45 minutes to 1 hour
White (navy)	45 minutes to 1¼ hours
Lentils	35 to 45 minutes (do not soak)
Split peas	45 minutes to 1 hour (do not soak)

cooking gluten-free whole grains

Free of EGG SOY NUT SUGAR OIL

When embarking on a gluten-free diet, variety, nutrition, and affordability are all important factors to consider. What makes a grain whole? It's when the bran and germ are still intact, thus providing vital nutrients like fiber and essential fats, vitamins, and minerals. By learning a few simple tips, you'll be able to rotate any number of grains into your diet.

TO CLEAN THE GRAINS: Rinse or soak them according to the directions below in cold water until the water runs clear. Drain in a fine-mesh strainer.

TO COOK THE GRAINS: Generally, grains are cooked in a two-part liquid to one-part grain ratio unless noted. Place the prepared grain in a saucepan with your liquid of choice—water, vegetable, chicken or beef stock, miso broth, or any type of seasoned liquid. Bring to a boil, cover, and reduce the heat to low. Simmer for the recommended time. Remove from the heat and allow the grain to rest for 5 minutes, fluff with a fork, and serve. Or cook rice in a rice cooker.

TO TOAST GRAINS: Not all grains benefit from toasting. For those that do, simply place the soaked or rinsed, well-strained grain in a saucepan over medium-high heat and toast, stirring frequently, until fragrant, about 5 minutes.

WHOLE GRAIN COOKING

1 Cup Grain	Method	Cooking Liquid	Time
Long-grain brown rice & Wehani	rinse and strain	2 cups	45 minutes
Short-grain brown rice	rinse and strain	2¼ cups	50 minutes
Red rice (Bhutan)	do not rinse	1¾ cups	25 minutes
Black rice (Forbidden)	do not rinse	1¾ cups	35 minutes
Wild rice	rinse and strain	3 cups	45 minutes
White rice (not a whole grain)	rinse optional	1¾ cups	20 minutes
Quinoa	soak, rinse, and strain	2 cups	20 minutes
Millet	rinse, strain, and toast	2 cups	15 to 20 minutes
Gluten-free steel-cut oat	rinse and strain	3 cups	30 minutes
Amaranth	rinse and strain	3 cups	25 to 30 minutes
Polenta	do not rinse	4 cups	40 minutes
Buckwheat toasted groats (kasha)	do not rinse	2½ cups	20 minutes

roasted peppers

Free of EGG SOY NUT SUGAR OIL

Charred food is generally not the desired result in cooking. However, when you're roasting peppers, charring the skin imparts a wonderful distinctive flavor to the flesh beneath. Here are four different methods that all work equally well, my favorite being the grill/barbecue method.

TO GRILL BELL PEPPER HALVES: Preheat a grill to 450°F (a hot fire). Cut the bell peppers in half lengthwise and remove the stems and seeds. Grill, skin-side down, until the skin is charred and bubbled. Turn and continue grilling the inside of the pepper for about 1 minute; do not blacken the inside. Transfer the peppers to a bowl, cover the bowl with a plate or plastic wrap, and allow the peppers to steam for about 20 minutes.

TO GRILL WHOLE PEPPERS, INCLUDING CHILES: Leave the peppers whole and place them on the hot grill, turning them until the skin is bubbled and completely charred. Transfer the peppers to a bowl, cover the bowl with a plate or plastic wrap, and allow the peppers to steam for about 20 minutes.

TO ROAST PEPPERS ON A GAS STOVE: Using tongs, set whole peppers over a gas flame, turning and watching constantly, until the skin bubbles and is completely charred on all sides. Transfer the peppers to a bowl, cover the bowl with a plate or with plastic wrap, and allow the peppers to steam for about 20 minutes.

TO ROAST PEPPERS UNDER A BROILER: Line the top rack of the oven with aluminum foil. Preheat the broiler. Cut the peppers in half lengthwise and remove the stems and seeds. Broil, skin-side up and about 3 inches from the heat source, until the skin bubbles and is completely charred. Transfer the peppers to a bowl, cover the bowl with a plate or with plastic wrap, and allow the peppers to steam for about 20 minutes.

TO CLEAN THE PEPPERS: Remove the charred skin by gently rubbing it off by hand or by lightly scraping it off with a sharp knife.

TO STORE THE PEPPERS: If you won't be using them immediately, cut the roasted, cleaned peppers into long segments and layer them in a dish with olive oil and any reserved juices. Cover the peppers tightly and refrigerate for up to 5 days.

grilled vegetables

SERVES 4 TO 6

Because the size of the vegetables can vary and different areas of the grill can be hotter than others, watch the grilling closely and use the suggested cooking times only as a guide. When making grilled vegetables for a large group, double or triple the recipe and grill the vegetables until they are well scored but still firm. Arrange them in a shallow roasting pan, cover tightly with aluminum foil, and place the pan in a 200°F oven for up to 45 minutes. The slow oven will finish steaming the vegetables and will give you the time you need to set up the rest of the food.

2 Japanese eggplants, unpeeled, and halved lengthwise

2 zucchini, unpeeled, and halved lengthwise

2 yellow crookneck squash, unpeeled, and halved lengthwise

2 red bell peppers, seeded, ribbed, and halved lengthwise

2 tablespoons olive oil

1 teaspoon salt

$1/2$ teaspoon freshly ground black pepper

2 teaspoons garlic powder

TO PREPARE AND GRILL THE VEGETABLES: Preheat the grill to 350°F (a medium-hot fire). Place the eggplant, zucchini, and yellow squash halves on a cutting board cut-side up. Using a small, sharp knife, score each vegetable half by making 3 to 4 diagonal slits, no more than $1/4$ to $1/2$-inch deep. Transfer the eggplant, zucchini, yellow squash, and bell pepper, cut-side up, to a large shallow roasting pan. Pour the olive oil over the vegetables and sprinkle with salt, pepper, and garlic powder. Using your hands, rub the oil and seasonings into the vegetables, coating them completely. Grill the vegetables, cut-side down, for about 6 minutes. Using tongs, turn the vegetables over so that the skin side is on the grill. Grill until the vegetables are tender, about 5 minutes longer. Arrange the grilled vegetables on a platter, cut-side up, and serve hot, warm, or cold.

grilled figs

Free of EGG SOY NUT SUGAR OIL

SERVES 4

When we installed our gas barbecue, we began grilling everything from appetizers to dessert—the dessert, of course, being fresh fruit. The first fruit we grilled was figs, and they were such a huge success that we've since tried numerous other fruits.

8 ripe black figs, rinsed and wiped dry

Preheat the grill to 350°F (a medium-hot fire) and lightly oil the grill racks. Cut each fig in half lengthwise. Grill the figs, cut-side down, for 2 minutes. Using tongs, turn the figs and grill until the figs are soft and caramelized, 3 to 4 minutes longer. Carefully transfer the figs to a plate, cut-side up. Allow the figs to cool to room temperature before serving, about 5 minutes.

grilled nectarines, peaches, *or apricots*

Free of EGG SOY NUT OIL

SERVES 4

4 unpeeled nectarines, peaches, or apricots

8 teaspoons light brown sugar (optional)

TO PREPARE AND GRILL THE FRUIT: Preheat the grill to 350°F (a medium-hot fire). Lightly oil the grill racks. Cut the fruit in half by cutting around the fruit down to the pit, following the natural seam. Separate the halves by rotating them in opposite directions, pulling them apart; remove and discard the pit. Grill the fruit, cut-side down, for about 3 minutes. Using tongs, turn the fruit over so that the cut side is up. In the hollow left by the pit, sprinkle each half with 1 teaspoon of brown sugar and grill for about 5 minutes longer. Carefully transfer the fruit to a plate, cut-side up. Allow the fruit to cool slightly, 3 to 4 minutes, before serving.

herb toast

Free of SOY NUT SUGAR

Herb Toast can be made up to 3 days ahead and stored at room temperature in tightly covered containers or heavy, plastic storage bags. Let the bread cool before storing or it will become soggy.

$1/3$ **cup olive oil**

4 cloves garlic, minced

1 tablespoon minced fresh rosemary

1 teaspoon minced fresh thyme

$1/4$ **teaspoon salt**

$1/8$ **teaspoon freshly ground black pepper**

1 loaf Fiber-Rich Sandwich Bread (page 137)

TO PREPARE THE BREAD: Preheat the oven to 250°F. Combine the olive oil, garlic, rosemary, thyme, salt, and pepper in a small saucepan and stir over low heat until fragrant, about 3 minutes. Slice the bread into $1/4$-inch-thick pieces. Using a pastry brush, lightly brush each of the slices with the olive oil mixture. Cut the bread lengthwise into 2-inch pieces or quarter into triangles, and place in a single layer on a baking sheet. Bake the bread until golden brown and crisp throughout, about 20 minutes. Check on the slices periodically, as they can burn easily. Transfer the toasts to a wire rack and cool completely.

gluten-free bread crumbs

Free of SOY NUT SUGAR OIL

MAKES 3 CUPS

1 loaf Fiber-Rich Sandwich Bread (page 137)

Preheat the oven to 300°F. Slice the bread into $1/2$-inch-thick slices and place in a single layer on a baking sheet. Bake until the bread is dry but not hard, 15 to 20 minutes. Remove from the oven and let cool. Break the slices up with your hands, then pulse in the blender or food processor until the texture ranges from fine to a little coarse. Cool completely and store at room temperature in a container with a tight-fitting lid for up to 5 days, or freeze for up to 2 weeks.

toasted nuts *and* seeds

Free of EGG SOY SUGAR OIL

Toasting nuts is a delicious way to bring out their crisp texture and full flavor. The method described here works equally well for shelled raw almonds, cashews, pine nuts, pecans, walnuts, and macadamia nuts. Nuts retain their heat long after being removed from the stove, so it is very important not to overcook them, because they will continue to darken as they cool.

TO TOAST NUTS: Place the nuts in a large skillet over medium-high heat. Toss them continuously in the skillet until the nuts begin to crackle and turn a light golden color. Transfer the nuts to a plate and spread them in a single layer to cool.

TO TOAST SESAME SEEDS: Place the seeds in a small skillet over medium-low heat. Toss the seeds continuously in the skillet until they begin to crackle and pop, 1 to 2 minutes. Transfer the seeds to a plate and spread them out in a single layer to cool.

TO ROAST NUTS: Preheat the oven to 300°F. Line the bottom of a rimmed baking sheet with parchment paper. Spread the nuts on the prepared pan in a single layer. Bake until they turn a light golden color, 10 to 15 minutes, depending on the size of the nuts. Nuts burn easily, so watch them closely.

TO STORE TOASTED OR ROASTED NUTS OR SEEDS: Allow the nuts or seeds to cool completely before you store them or they will become soggy. Store in an airtight container at room temperature for up to 1 week.

savory nuts

MAKES 4 CUPS

I find myself baking up a batch of these nuts every week—they've become a staple in our home. When my energy begins to dip in the afternoon, I'll grab a small handful of these nuts for a quick pick-me-up. I particularly like mixing them with raw nuts and dried cranberries, or raisins and will sometimes even toss in a bit of dried sea palm—a sea vegetable—which makes for a very tasty and healthy treat.

1 cup raw shelled whole almonds (5 ounces)

1 cup raw shelled walnut halves (5 ounces)

1 cup raw shelled pecan halves (5 ounces)

1 cup shelled whole cashews (5 ounces)

1 tablespoon Bragg Liquid Aminos or gluten-free tamari

TO PREPARE THE NUTS: Preheat the oven to 325°F. Combine the almonds, walnuts, pecans, and cashews in a large bowl; toss to combine. Add the Braggs and toss to coat.

Spread the nuts in a single layer on a nonstick jelly-roll pan. Bake for 12 minutes on the first side then using a spatula turn the nuts over. Continue baking for an additional 8 to 10 minutes. Nuts can burn easily so watch them closely; bake until they turn a rich golden color.

Remove the pan from the oven and allow to cool for about 10 minutes. Loosen the nuts with a spatula and cool completely in the pan for about two hours.

TO STORE THE NUTS: It is important that the nuts are cooled completely before storage or they will become soft. Store the nuts in an airtight container at room temperature for 1 week.

candied pecans

MAKES 2¹/₂ CUPS

These nuts can be used in a variety of ways. They make a nice accompaniment to an hors d'oeuvre table, or they can be tossed into a salad or used as a dessert topping. For a hot and spicy variation, add ¹/₄ teaspoon cayenne pepper and ¹/₂ teaspoon each of ground cinnamon, ginger, and allspice to the sugar before adding it to the egg white. If you prefer, use walnuts instead of the pecans.

1 large egg white

¹/₈ teaspoon salt

¹/₂ cup sugar

2¹/₂ cups shelled pecan halves (10 ounces)

2 tablespoons canola oil

TO COAT THE PECANS: Using an electric mixer, beat the egg white and salt in a large bowl until foamy. Gradually add the sugar, beating just until blended. Do not overbeat; the mixture should be runny. Add the pecan halves and stir to coat with a rubber spatula.

TO BAKE THE PECANS: Preheat the oven to 325°F. Distribute the oil evenly on a nonstick rimmed baking sheet. Spread the pecans on the prepared pan in a single layer, separating any that stick together. Bake for 10 minutes on the first side and then, using a spatula, turn the pecans over, separating any that stick together. Continue baking until they turn a rich golden color, 8 to 10 minutes longer. Nuts can burn easily, so watch them closely. Total baking time is about 20 minutes.

Remove the pan from the oven and allow the pecans to cool for about 10 minutes. Loosen them with a spatula and cool completely in the pan for about 2 hours.

Cool the pecans completely before storing them, or they will become soft. Store the pecans in an airtight container at room temperature for up to 1 week.

date syrup *and* orange date syrup

Free of EGG SOY NUT SUGAR OIL

MAKES 2 CUPS

The high sugar content of dates yields a very tasty syrup that is rich in potassium and a good source of iron, magnesium, copper, niacin, and fiber. Orange pairs very nicely with dates and adds additional sweetness to the syrup with subtle orange flavor.

DATE SYRUP

1¼ to 1½ cups filtered cold water

1 cup pitted medjool dates, halved (12 to 14 dates)

1 teaspoon freshly squeezed lemon juice

ORANGE DATE SYRUP

1½ cups freshly squeezed orange juice (about 3 oranges)

1 cup pitted medjool dates, halved (12 to 14 dates)

TO PREPARE BOTH SYRUPS: In a blender, combine all of the ingredients. Cover the blender and pulse the mixture a few times to break up the fruit. Whirl at top speed, occasionally scraping down the sides, until the mixture is smooth and creamy, about 2 minutes. Transfer the syrup to a glass container with a tight-fitting lid, label it with the date, and refrigerate for up to 2 weeks. Before using, stir the syrup to blend.

bibliography

Brostoff, Jonathan, MD. and Linda Gamlin. *Food Allergies & Food Intolerance, .* Rochester, VT: Healing Arts Press, 2000.

Campbell, Colin T., MD. *The China Study*. Dallas, TX: BenBella Books Inc., 2006.

Case, Shelley, RD. *Gluten-Free Diet, 8th Edition*. Regina, Canada: Case Nutrition Consulting Inc., 2010.

Carter, Jill, with Alison Edwards. *Allergy Exclusion Diet*. Carlsbad, CA: Hay House, Inc., 2003.

Cheetham, Grace. *A Cook's Bible Gluten-Free, Wheat-Free & Dairy-Free Recipes*. London, UK: Duncan Baird Publishers Ltd., 2009.

Cupillard, Valérie. *Gluten-Free Gourmet Desserts and Baked Goods*. Summertown,TN: Book Publishing Company, 2006.

Esselstyn, Rip. *The Engine 2 Diet*. New York, NY: Wellness Central, 2009.

Fleming, Alisa Marie. *Go Dairy Free*. Henderson, NV: Fleming Ink, 2008.

Fuhrman, Joel, MD. *Eat For Health*. Flemington, NJ: Gift of Health Press, 2010.

Haynes, Antony J. and Antoinette, Savill. *The Food Intolerance Bible*. San Francisco, CA: Harper Thorsons, 2005.

Joneja, Janice Vickerstaff. *Dealing with Food Allergies*. Boulder, CO: Bull Publishing Co., 2003.

Lowell, Jax Peters. *The Gluten-Free Bible*. New York: Owl Books, 2005.

Page, Linda. *Healthy Healing, 12th Edition*. Carmel Valley, CA: Healthy Healing Publications, 2004.

Pulde, Alona, MD, and Lederman, Matthew, MD. *Keep It Simple, Keep It Whole*. Los Angeles, CA: Exsalus Health & Wellness Center, 2009.

Walsh, William E., MD. *Food Allergies*. New York, NY: John Wiley & Sons, 2000.

Shurtleff, William, and Akiko Aoyagi. *The Book of Tofu*. Berkeley, CA: Ten Speed Press, 2001.

Wittenberg, Margaret M. *New Good Food*. Berkeley: Ten Speed Press, 2007.

resources

Government Agencies and Food Resources

American Academy of Allergy
Asthma & Immunology
800-822-2762
www.aaaai.org

Food and Drug Administration (FDA)
Freedom of Information Staff
888-463-6332
www.fda.gov

The Food Allergy and Anaphylaxis
Network (FAAN)
800-929-4040
www.foodallergy.org

The National Institute of Allergy
and Infectious Diseases (NIAID)
NIAID Office of Communications
and Government Relations
866-284-4107
www.niaid.nih.gov

National Osteoporosis Foundation
800-223-9994 or 202-223-2226
www.nof.org

U.S. Food and Drug Administration
"Living With Food Allergies" by
Anne Munoz-Furlong *FDA Consumer
Magazine*, July/August 2001, Volume
35, Number 4

U.S. Department of Agriculture
(USDA)
Nutrient Data Laboratory/
Agricultural Research Service/
Beltsville Human Nutrition
Research Center
301-504-0630
www.ars.usda.gov./ba/bhnrc/ndl

U.S. Soyfoods Directory
www.soyfoods.com

Nutrition and Recipe Online Resources

Living Without Magazine
http;//www.livingwithout.com

Whole Foods Market
www.wholefoodsmarket.com/
healthstartshere
www.wholefoodsmarket.com/meat/
welfare.php

World's Healthiest Foods
www.whfoods.org

Gluten-Free Information

American Celiac Disease Alliance
703-622-3331
www.americanceliac.org

American Celiac Society
504-737-3293
www.americanceliacsociety.org

Celiac Disease Foundation
818-990-2354
www.celiac.org

Gluten-Free, Casein-Free
*Dietary Intervention for Autistic
Spectrum Disorders*
www.gfcfdiet.com

The Gluten Intolerance Group
253-833-6655
www.gluten.net

Gluten-Free Vacation Information
www.bobandruths.com

Allergy-Friendly Dining Out Online
Support/*The Essential Gluten-Free
Restaurant Guide*
www.triumphdining.com

Welcoming Guests with Food
Allergies
www.foodallergy.org

*Let's Eat Out with Celiac/Coeliac and
Food Allergies*
www.glutenfreepassport.com

Online Discussion Board Support
www.glutenfreeforum.com

Seafood Sustainability

Monterey Bay Seafood Watch Program
www.montereybayaquarium.org/cr/seafoodwatch.aspx

Marine Stewardship Council
www.msc.org

Blue Ocean Institute
www.blueocean.org

Complementary and Alternative Medical Practices

Institute for Functional Medicine
www.functionalmedicine.org

U.S. Center for Complementary and Alternative Medicine
www.nccam.nih.gov

Comprehensive Labs/Celiac Genetics Testing

Prometheus Laboratories Inc.
888-423-5227, option 3
www.prometheuslabs.com

Kimball Genetics
800-320-1807
www.kimballgenetics.com

Mayo Medical Laboratories
800-423-5227
www.mayomedicallaboratories.com

Manufacturers and Distributors

Applegate Farms
Dairy- and gluten-free sausages, hot dogs, bacon, and cold cuts
800-358-8289
www.applegatefarms.com

Bob's Red Mill Natural Foods, Inc.
Gluten-free flours, oats, grains, mixes, flax and chia seeds, xanthan and guar gum
800-349-2173
www.bobsredmill.com

Bragg Live Foods, Inc.
Apple cider vinegar, Bragg Liquid Aminos
800-446-1990
www.bragg.com

Cascade Fresh, Inc.
Amande cultured almond milk yogurt
800-511-0057
www.cascadefresh.com

Daiya Foods, Inc.
Dairy-, gluten-, soy-, and nut-free cheese alternatives
877-324-9211
www.daiyafoods.com

Discount Natural Foods, Inc.
Tribest Yolife dairy-free yogurt starter
888-392-9237
www.healthytraders.com

Double Rainbow Gourmet Ice Creams, Inc.
Soy cream frozen desserts
800-489-3580
www.doublerainbow.com

Earth Balance
Vegan, gluten-free, and soy alternative spread (butter and margarine substitute), nonhydrogenated, nonGMO
201-421-3970
www.earthbalancenatural.com

Eden Foods, Inc.
Milk alternatives (not all are GF), beans, 100% buckwheat pasta, all organic
888-424-3336
www.edenfoods.com

Enjoy Life Foods
Chocolate chips, multi-allergy dairy-, casein-, gluten-, peanut-, soy-, and egg-free products
888-503-6569
www.enjoylifefoods.com

Follow Your Heart
Dairy- and gluten-free Vegenaise, cream cheese, sour cream, and cheese alternatives
818-725-2820
www.followyourheart.com

Food Directions, Inc.
Tinkayáda gluten- and dairy-free pastas and bread products
888-323-2388
www.tinkyada.com

Food for Life Baking Co., Inc.
Gluten- and dairy-free English muffins and bread products
800-797-5090
www.foodforlife.com

Galaxy Nutritional Foods
Vegan soy and rice cheese alternatives, dairy- and gluten-free
800-441-9419
www.galaxyfoods.com

GI ProHealth
Dairy-free yogurt starter
877-219-3559
www.giprohealth.com

Gifts of Nature, Inc.
Gluten-free safe oats
888-275-0003
www.giftsofnature.net

Gluten-Free Mall
Wide assortment of gluten-free products
866-575-3720
www.glutenfreemall.com

Gluten-Free Pantry
Wide assortment of gluten-free online products
860-633-3826
www.glutenfree.com

Grainaissance, Inc.
Dairy- and gluten-free products, Amazake beverages, rice nog, pudding, and mochi
800-472-4697
www.grainaissance.com

Häagen-Dazs/Ice Cream Partners
Assorted sorbets
800-767-0120
www.haagen-daz.com

Hain Celestial Group, Inc.
Distributors of dairy-free and
gluten-free product lines, including:
Arrowhead Mills, DeBoles, Hain Pure
Foods, Imagine Foods, Spectrum
expeller pressed oils, and Sunspire
chocolate chips
800-434-4246
www.hain-celestial.com

Kinnikinnick Foods, Inc.
Gluten- and dairy-free bread products,
and graham crackers
877-503-4466
www.kinnikinnick.com

Knudsen and Sons, Inc.
Fruit juices and spreads
888-569-6993
www.rwknudsenfamily.com

La Tortilla Factory Sonoma
Gluten-free teff flour tortilla wraps
800-446-1516
www.latortillafactory.com

Lundberg Family Farms
Rice and grain products
530-882-4551
www.lundberg.com

Manitoba Harvest
Hemp milk alternative, protein,
and seed
800-665-4367
www.manitobaharvest.com

Morinaga Nutritional Foods, Inc.
Mori-Nu silken-style tofu
800-699-8638
www.morinu.com

Nutraceutical Corporation
Nutritional yeast flakes
800-669-8877
www.nutraceutical.com

Nancy's Springfield Creamery
Cultured soy yogurt
541-689-2911
www.nancysyogurt.com

Now Foods
Stevia (liquid and powder), nutritional
yeast flakes, agar agar, spirulina,
chlorella
888-669-3663
www.nowfoods.com

Pacific Foods of Oregon, Inc.
Milk alternatives, and chicken and
vegetable stock
503-692-9666
www.pacificfoods.com

Pulmuone Wildwood, Inc.
Organic sprouted tofu, soy milk,
soy yogurt
800-499-8638
www.pulmuonewildwood.com

Ricera Foods
Organic Rice Yogurt
707-824-0119
www.ricerafoods.com

Rudi's Organic Bakery
Gluten-free certified breads
877-293-0876
www.rudisbakery.com

San-J International, Inc.
Gluten-free Tamari soy sauce and
stir-fry sauces
800-446-5500
www.san-j.com

Scharffen Berger and Dagoba
Organic Chocolate
Baking chocolate
866-608-6944
www.artisanconfection.com

Tofutti Brands, Inc.
Dairy-free frozen desserts, sour cream,
and cream cheese
908-272-2400
www.tofutti.com

Turtle Mountain Inc.
Frozen desserts: Organic So Delicious,
Purely Decadent Dairy-Free, Purely
Decadent Coconut Milk, It's Soy
Delicious, So Delicious Coconut Water
Sorbet, Sweet Nothings, and So
Delicious Coconut Milk beverage
866-388-7853
www.turtlemountain.com

Udi's Gluten-Free Foods
Gluten-Free certified breads, muffins,
granola, and pizza crust
303-657-1600
www.udisglutenfree.com

Vance's Foods
DariFree powdered potato milk
alternative
800-497-4834
www.vancesfoods.com

Vitasoy USA, Inc.
Nasoya tofu, milk alternatives, and
Azumaya products (wonton wraps)
800-328-8638
www.vitasoy-usa.com

White Wave, Inc.
Silk soy milk creamer, yogurt, and soy
nog; White Wave tofu and tempeh
800-488-9283
www.whitewave.com

Whole Foods Market, Inc.
Natural and organic food supermarkets
(USA, Canada, and United Kingdom),
complete assortment of natural and
organic foods and beverages, including
an extensive offering of dairy- and
gluten-free products
512-477-4455
www.wholefoodsmarket.com

WholeSoy & Co.
Organic soy yogurt, dairy- and
gluten-free
877-569-6376
www.wholesoyco.com

index

the **dairy-free** and **gluten-free** kitchen

the **dairy-free** and **gluten-free** kitchen

about the author

Denise Jardine is a certified nutrition educator, an author, and an engaging speaker. She works at Whole Foods Market®, Northern California, as the Regional Healthy Eating Program Coordinator delivering lively presentations to businesses, hospitals, health-care providers, seniors, and schools all over the northern part of the state. Her expertise has become increasingly focused on special dietary needs, food allergies, and food sensitivities, and how to address them in holistic ways as these issues become ever more prevalent in the mainstream population. Denise lives in the San Francisco Bay Area with her husband Robert. For more, visit www.dairyfreeglutenfreekitchen.com.

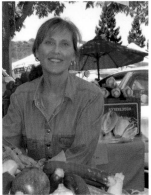

photo by Robert Jardine

The information contained in this book is based on the experience and research of the author. It is not intended as a substitute for consulting with your physician or other health-care provider. Any attempt to diagnose and treat an illness should be done under the direction of a health-care professional. The publisher and author are not responsible for any adverse effects or consequences resulting from the use of any of the suggestions, preparations, or procedures discussed in this book.

Published in the United States by Ten Speed Press,
an imprint of the Crown Publishing Group,
a division of Random House, Inc., New York.
www.crownpublishing.com
www.tenspeed.com

This book was originally published in the United States under the title *Recipes for Dairy-Free Living* by Celestial Arts Publishing, an imprint of Ten Speed Press, Berkeley, 2001.

The essay on pages 6–7, "Calcium 101" copyright ©2000 by Kazuko Aoyagi

Ten Speed Press and the Ten Speed Press colophon are registered trademarks of Random House, Inc.

Library of Congress Cataloging-in-Publication Data
Jardine, Denise.
The dairy-free & gluten-free kitchen / Denise Jardine; photography by Caroline Kopp and Erin Kunkel.
        p. cm.
Includes index.
1. Milk-free diet—Recipes. 2. Gluten-free diet—Recipes.
3. Food allergy. 4. Cookbooks. I. Title.
RM234.5.J373 2011
641.3—dc23
                                2011027420
ISBN 978-1-60774-224-1

Printed in China

Cover and text design by Toni Tajima
Cover photographs by Erin Kunkel, except for
back cover, top right photograph by Caroline Kopp
Food styling for Erin Kunkel photographs by Erin Quon
Food styling for Caroline Kopp photographs by Pouké

10 9 8 7 6
Revised Edition